Foreword by
World's #1 Motivational Speaker

M000208641

The Handbook to™

Holistic Health

H³

A Self-help Guide to Live
HAPPY, HEALTHY
and WEALTHY.

LOCAL EXPERTS GROUP

Local Experts Group
1111 Finch Ave West #401
Toronto Ontario Canada M3J 2E5
647.919.8131
www.localexpertsgroup.com

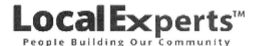

People Building Our Community

Disclaimer

We have tried to work very hard to ensure this book brings you best practices in the field of holistic health. However, the contents of this book should be used for information only. Medical concerns must be directed to your primary medical practitioner. The coauthors, affiliate organizations and publishers assume no responsibility for any decision made as a result of reading this book that can affect your business or personal life.

Unless otherwise indicated, Scripture quotations taken from the King James Version (KJV) - public domain.

Scripture quotations taken from the Holy Bible, New Living translation (NTL). Copyright ©1996, 2004, 2007by Tyndale House Foundation. Used by permission of Tyndale House Publishers Inc.

2nd Printing
Printed in Canada

ISBN: 978-1-9995358-0-3

Table of Contents

Dedication

We, the Coauthors, collectively dedicate this book to you, the reader. Thank you for investing in your continued education and for seeking out authentic material. Now that you are reading this, we hope you will apply the portions relevant to you. Please think of a family member and/or a friend who can also benefit from this book. You are welcome to keep this book in your private collection, and we also suggest you gift or lend it to someone who needs to see this material. Again, this is for you and if you have any questions or concerns, you will find our contact information at the end of each chapter. For a free chapter or to order additional copies at a discounted rate, be sure to visit H3Book.com

Endorsement

The information presented in this book satisfied the requirement of the World Organization of Natural Medicine Education Department. This endorsement is a symbol of recognition of the promotion of humanitarian values through education. We have hereby ascribed and affixed the seal of the organization, www.wonm.org.

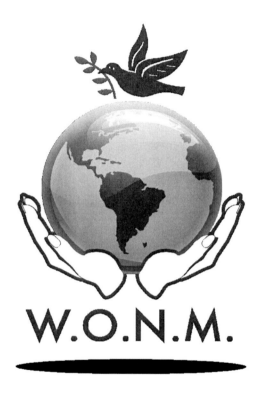

Acknowledgements

This book has been a dream of mine and now you hold the finished copy in your hands. What started out as a small project has now turned into something, I am so proud of. So many people contributed to this book that it is hard to know where to start. This is a true product of The Power of Collaboration™.

First of all, I would like to acknowledge the leadership of Her Majesty The Queen, His Holiness Pope Francis, Prime Minister Justin Trudeau, Prime Minister Theresa May, President Donald Trump, President David A. Granger, Prime Minister Narendra Modi and all other world leaders for their dedication to serving humanity.

I acknowledge virtual mentors namely; Oprah Winfrey, Warren Buffet, Sir Richard Branson, Bill Gates, Dr. Oz, Dr. Phil, Ellen DeGeneres, Tony Robbins, Dr. Brian Tracy, Bob Proctor, Jack Canfield, Dr. Nido Qubein, Dr. Sanjay Gupta, Dr. Deepak Chopra, Grant Cardone, Naveen Jain, Steve Harvey, Priyanka Chopra, Will Smith, Aubrey Drake Graham, Lilly Singh and most importantly, Mr. Les Brown.

To all my amazing co-authors; thank you so much for sharing your knowledge so freely. Each one of you shared from the heart and truly gave your best. This book wouldn't be possible if it weren't for you.

Dr. Ona Brown, thanks to you and your team at *World Impact Now™*, for seeing the scope of this project and how much it is going to help others and joining us on this journey. Your chapter, of you and your Dad, Mr. Les Brown, shows how Holistic Medicine played a vital role in his healing and will encourage so many others.

To, Dame Dr. Sheila McKenzie and your organization *World Organization of Natural Medicine Clinics for Humanity™*. Thank you for endorsing, collaborating and co-authoring with me on this project.

Prof. Dr. George Grant; Founder of the *International Academy of Wellness™*. Thank you for your continued support, inspiration and vision as my Health and Wellness mentor, co-author and Guru Dad.

To Raymond Aaron and Sunil Tulsiani, thank you for showing me what is possible in this world. You are both amazing mentors and I have learned so much from you both. Your belief in me has allowed me to propel forward at an incredible speed.

A special thanks to my parents and sisters. You've watched me grow and have been there to encourage me all the way. I wouldn't be who I was if it weren't for you.

I want to thank my team at LocalExpertsGroup.com for the amazing work you are doing in publishing "The Handbook to™" series of books.

I want to thank you, the reader. Books like these, only become valuable as others buy it, read it and apply what is in it. You are on the fantastic journey of life and I hope this book, helps you to live a more fulfilled one.

Last, but most certainly not least, is my wife, Divya. You share my heart and you encourage me to go after my dreams. My life would be incomplete without you. Your support made this book possible. Not only did you contribute a chapter to this book, but you gave up time with me, so I could make this collaborative book a reality. You are the joy of my heart, thank you seven billion times!!!

God Bless., Raymond Harlall
Publisher & Producer

Introduction

Everyone has a choice when it comes to their health and well-being. Most people ignore it until something bad happens and then they scramble to try and get it back. There are the few who take it seriously and realize if they want to live a long life they need to act now and not wait until sickness and disease arrives. Which one are you?

The second choice has to do with what route you choose. I am so thankful for the doctors and the work they do. They save lives every day. Most doctors truly care about their patients and want to do what is best for them and I applaud them for it.

But . . .

There is much they do not know or consider as options. There is a whole world of alternative methods out there which are sometimes more effective than traditional medicine. Doctors are not taught these methods and have given them a bad rap because they don't understand their power.

Holistic Lifestyle

This book is going to teach you how to live holistically, or maybe a better way to spell it would be 'wholistically'. Holistic is defined on Dictionary.com as:

> Incorporating the concept of holism, or the idea that the whole is more than merely the sum of its parts, in theory, or practice.

It is looking at your whole life and making sure all the parts are in balance. It is coming to the realization every part of you affects the other. They are interdependent and you cannot live a full life without all of them working well together.

This includes your mind, body and spirit. It's about having a healthy body full of energy and vigour. A mind that can handle any situation thrown at it and is peaceful and happy. A spirit that knows there is Someone or something more which guides you and has a plan. When you combine all three, you will live the life of your dreams. Isn't this what you want?

This Book Contains It All

In this book are twenty experts in holistic living, who have shared their knowledge freely with you. Each chapter will focus in on a specific part, whether it be mind, body or spirit:

If you are interested in the physical side of holistic health, be sure to read the chapters written by: Dr. Ona Brown, Prof. Dr. George Grant, Dr. Sheila McKenzie, Mr. Charles Tchoreret, Cheryl Ivaniski, Dr. Akbar Khan, Prof. Dr. Stanley Ngui, Ms. Josephine Marcellin, Ms. Maricel Gonzales and Ms. Tiffanie Carr.

The great thing is these ideas are not hard to implement. Pick a chapter, read through it and start out by doing one thing they suggest. Each week if you incorporate one teaching you will find your life changed in the next year. What have you got to lose? Just try it!

I decided to approach each of these co-authors to help me with this book because I saw so many people struggling when they didn't need to. You have options beyond the traditional routes. You can see yourself whole and learn how to balance all parts of you in equal harmony.

If you are interested in your mental and spiritual health, then you want to read the chapters written by: Mr. Benjamin Stone, Ms. Cora Cristobal, Ms. Divya Sieudarsan, Ms. Hailey Patry, Master Teresa Yeung, Mr. James MacNeil, Mr. Jim Hetherington, Mr. Raymond Young & Ms. Hailee Young, Dr. Sany Seifi and my chapter.

These experts live what they teach. They are experts in education and experience and they take what they do seriously. Each one has shared not only their knowledge, but their heart as well. They want to see you happy and whole. But this can only happen if you take action.

I know you want a better life. You wouldn't be reading this book unless you did. The best thing to do is follow the guidance each of these experts has provided. They studied and learned and have chosen the best course of action for themselves. Not everything in this book applies to you, but when you find what does, don't just put the book down and think, "I will get to this next week." Start now with one small action that you can do today. Your body, mind and soul will thank you years down the road.

I am so thankful I made the change and I know you will be too. My deepest thoughts are for you to have a life that is everything you want your life to be. So, come on, join me on this journey into holistic health and see what it can do for you.

To a Life of So Much More,

Raymond Harlall
Co-Founder of *Local Experts Group*

Foreword
By: Les Brown

I am a person who loves life...and each day I wake up with excitement because I am committed to living my dreams with passion until I exit this thing called life. Which has me in a constant state of discovery to uncover the various ways to 'live full and die empty.'

Both traditional and non-traditional/holistic medicine were contributing factors to me becoming a sickness conqueror. I won't share all the details with you here, as my daughter, Ona, did a wonderful job of telling our story in her chapter of this great book. However, I encourage you to dive into this much-needed information with a sense of urgency . . . as if your life depended on it -- because it does.

Socrates once said that, "An undisciplined life . . . is an insane life!" I encourage people to take their health seriously and become more disciplined . . . because for quite some time I did not. For most of my career, I truly believed that I could eat whatever I wanted, as much as I wanted, push my body to its limits with unending travel and reap no consequences for my choices . . . and I was totally wrong.

Once you decide to pursue your greatness, you must become responsible for all areas of your life. You cannot control what life throws your way, but you can control who you are committed to being in the midst of the inevitable tough times of life.

I had a friend that I had been encouraging to publish her writings. She had written books and poems and never acted on sharing them with the world. I spoke to her about it many times. At last, I convinced her not to wait any longer and she agreed that it was finally time. The next day, I got news from her husband that she had died unexpectedly! When I visited her house, I found stacks of unfinished projects written by her that could have helped so many and now the world will never know of her work.

LET'S LEARN FROM THIS STORY!! IT IS AN EXAMPLE OF WHY WE MUST LIVE EACH DAY TO THE FULLEST!!

In my journey back to health, I realized that if I was going to fight cancer and stay alive, I was going to have to incorporate more than just traditional medicine. In order to stay strong physically, I was going to have to stay strong mentally, emotionally and spiritually as well. I utilized various holistic therapies to create an environment where the whole of me could be healed.

Some of the doctors I saw said that I was going to die. I said, "NO WAY. I AM GOING TO LIVE! I am going to continue on because there are greater works for me to do on this earth!!"

I am so happy for this collaboration between my daughter Ona Brown and Raymond Harlall. You are going to learn many strategies in this book to heal your body, stay healthy holistically and how to keep your mind and spirit strong in the process.

Don't wait for tragedy to strike before you take your health seriously. Be proactive, adhere to the recommended action steps by the experts in this book. When I was young, I was motivated to action by the threat of a switch on my behind by my adopted mother, Miss Mamie Brown. As I got older, I came to understand that motivation has to come from within . . . especially when you endure a whopping by life. Take your health seriously and may you live a full, long life that provides you with more than enough time for the world to behold the GREATNESS that is within YOU . . . because it is your responsibility to BRING IT OUT!

Les Brown
The Motivator/Mamie Brown's Baby Boy

Chapter 1

Rising Above the Storms of Life

By: Dr. Ona Brown

Have you ever experienced a time of back-to-back blows when you felt like life would not give you an opportunity to catch your breath or even get your bearings? My father, Les Brown and I went through a difficult period like that. We learned a lot and grew closer as a family. I am grateful for all of the wisdom, knowledge and strength that was gained as a result. In this chapter, I am going to share our story with the intention of encouraging someone who may find themselves or someone they love facing their own turbulent storm.

The First Blow

I can remember when I first joined Dad's company. Most people might have assumed I would get a high-level position, but my dad knew better. What would I learn if I started at the top? I would never understand true success if everything was handed to me, so I started out at an entry-level position as a receptionist. I also volunteered to handle all of the correspondence that came into the Les Brown Unlimited office. (It was a time when people actually mailed letters via the postal service.) We received hundreds of heartfelt letters on a weekly basis.

My father had thousands of devoted followers and fans, even before social media, who wanted to express their love and appreciation and share how much he had touched their lives. So, I took charge of managing that huge project. I created a system for customizing form letters, which we tweaked to each specific person and had my father sign whenever he was in town.

When you are faithful to the little things, bigger opportunities will eventually become available. Over time, I started negotiating my father's contractual agreements and was able to secure higher-paying engagements for him. I managed his very first highest-paid international contract. Then I started working with the speaker bureaus and re-establishing our relationships with them. I was the quiet power behind the scenes of his vision. I loved supporting my dad while also discovering the beauty of the self-development world that was slowly becoming my magnificent obsession.

This was during the early '90s, when our family business became increasingly busier, sometimes booking twenty to thirty events in one month. Les Brown the Motivator could easily be in New York on Monday, Los Angeles on Tuesday and perhaps London, England on Wednesday. Sometimes there were even two events in one day. Mr. Les Brown was in

3

such huge demand around the world and we were conducting business at a breathless pace . . . it was literally non-stop.

One day my father was on the radio discussing prostate-cancer awareness and telling men about the importance of booking a prostate exam. He said on air, "It's not right for me to tell men to do things that I'm not willing to do myself, even though I would rather not do this."

He moved forward on getting a prostate examination and that was when an unexpected blow came. He was diagnosed with prostate cancer.

That news flipped our whole world upside down. How could this be? My dad is so strong, so vibrant. He's invincible, he's my hero and now, instead of enjoying life, we are asked to make treatment decisions we were unprepared to make. Prostate removal? Radiation-seed implants? Chemotherapy?

We opted for the radiation-seed implants and as much holistic healing as possible. He went to several holistic institutes that helped him to design a plan to win the battle of cancer. I knew deep down inside that if my dad was going to win, I was going to have to help him as much as possible. I invited him to live with me during this time and moved him into my master bedroom, so we could make it a healing space of peace and hope.

But that's when the next series of blows came. By this point, the radiation-seed implants had been inserted and he was bedridden most of the time and in a lot of pain. His best friend since third grade, Uncle Boo, who was his business partner and would help him on the road, passed away waiting on a liver transplant. His mother, my grandmother, Ms. Mamie Brown, also departed from this thing called life. Finally, he went through a very public divorce from someone he loved dearly. Just a few of the major hits we took as a family within a short range of time; perhaps less than six to eight months of unexpected challenges.

Dad was determined he was going to live. It wasn't easy. We had to literally take it one day at a time. It felt like every day was a continuation of a death-defying fight. I knew we had to be strong together. There were brief moments when the doubts would come and we would have to battle them. Our resolve would grow stronger with each challenge we faced.

4

We were fighting daily to feed life into his cells in various ways by juicing organic fruits and vegetables every day and playing peaceful music and inspirational messages. We kept healing music playing in the background, like you might hear in a spa — music that was very soothing to both the cells and the soul. For inspirational words, we would put on Dr. Norman Vincent Peal, Bishop TD Jakes, Jim Rohn and Dr. Wayne Dyer, just to name a few. I even played some of Dad's recordings to reinforce, inside of him, his own beliefs.

We focused on various dimensions of healing for him: the physical, the mental and the spiritual. If he was going to defeat this, we could not take a one-sided approach . . . it all had to be taken care of and with a sense of urgency.

I also did my best to talk to Dad in a very loving, supportive way that spoke life into him. I would say, "You're going to get through this, Dad. We are just in the eye of a storm. We have been teaching this nationally and around the world. Now it's time for us to live the message we bring and know that we are going to make it through this together."

When Your Belief Is Tested

The doctors said, "Mr. Brown, we've examined you and unfortunately the radiation-seed implant treatments have not had the effect we had hoped for." They said, "You might as well get your affairs in order, because with the amount of cancer that is still in you, we are giving you a three to five-year prognosis."

That was a hard hit.

We had to press forward with our efforts, discipline and hard work. We were fully aware that this was not about just feeding life to the cells and creating a healthy environment, but also dealing with the battlefield of the mind. Pouring into and nurturing his mind was imperative for us to stay the course.

We would read positive, healing books. We strongly believe in the power of the spoken word. Knowing that words have power, Dad would repeat empowering affirmations about being a cancer conqueror.

Powerful statements such as "I am BIGGER than ANY CHALLENGE that I am facing. I am HEALED, WHOLE and COMPLETE . . . and cancer-FREE! I AM HEALTHY and HAPPY!

Or...

"I give THANKS that I am CANCER FREE and my MIND, BODY and SPIRIT are TOTALLY and COMPLETELY HEALED!!!!

I am COMMITTED, CONSISTENT and DEDICATED to maintaining SPIRITUAL, OPTIMUM HEALTH, ENERGY and WELL-BEING. I thank GOD, I am TOTALLY and COMPLETELY HEALED!!!"

Research was also something we found to be encouraging. We knew that if someone else had been able to defeat various forms of cancer—what Dad called the little c—then there was more hope for our victory as well.

We found out about Dr. Day. She was given a very short prognosis of two to three years because she had a tumour in her breast the size of a lemon. The doctors wanted to do several procedures and she decided that she would go about it holistically.

She walked and got sunlight every day. She stayed away from all negativity. She found out through her research that laughter was extremely healing and good for the body. She loved The Three Stooges comedy show and she would watch it every day to bring laughter into her life, which boosts the immune system. Dr. Day lived way beyond her expected two to three-year prognosis.

With that, I started making sure that Dad laughed every day and that we walked whenever he could, even if it was only for a block. He got sunlight every day, even if he just sat on the porch or the balcony. Whatever we had to do to get him into those things that she said were a powerful combination of healing, we did.

Reading, listening to positive materials, laughter and keeping to a diet of mostly highly nutritional raw foods and juices, with a little bit of protein every now and then as a big treat, made a difference.

I did catch him one time, at about 2 in the morning, with a chicken wing in his mouth. I said, "Daddy, put down the chicken wing and back away; it's not worth it. Help me to help you."
He replied, "I just wanted a little, tiny taste of chicken . . . do you think this is a form of sleep walking?" Sometimes, you just have to laugh.

Three years later the doctors were scratching their heads and saying, "You should have been gone by now. How are you still here? You are a walking miracle; it looks like your cancer is in remission. Your PSA [prostate specific antigen] is very low. Congratulations, Mr. Brown." Dad actually renamed the medical term P.S.A. to give it a new meaning for him personally . . . Positively Staying Alive!

It was a beautiful and exciting time. Even now I look at him in amazement, because I know there were periods where he was bedridden and in a lot of pain and we didn't know if he would make it.

Just When You Think Life Is Getting Better
When he resumed his professional speaking engagements, some challenges and pain remained, yet he was still able to motivate an audience of thousands. To witness someone, stand and be in pain all the way to the microphone and then be transformed into this vessel that is so energetic and inspirational amazed me beyond words.

There he was in this powerful place and people were getting fired up, people were crying and I'm bawling, because I'm wondering how this man can exhibit so much love for people and uplift them in the midst of his own aches and struggles.

It was magical and miraculous. Afterwards, he would say, "I don't even know what happened. Once I started speaking, the pain just went away; I didn't feel anything."

I would say, "Because when you walk in your purpose, you step into a different dimension of existence and being."

My dad getting through cancer gave us the ability and the strength to know that we didn't have to buy into anyone else's opinion about what the future holds. We all have the ability to rise above our fears if we are willing to do what is required and to focus on in-depth healing and the possibilities of life.

So many things have happened since then. We learned that my father also had some blockages in his heart, so he ended up having six stints put in. Next, he was told he had cancer in seven different areas of his spine.

He said, "Did you say seven areas? I'm so glad to hear that."

The doctor, dumbfounded, said, "What? Are you kidding me? Why do you say that?"

Dad replied, "Because seven is my lucky number. I was born on February 17th; my telephone number begins with 702 and the Bible says the Israelites walked around the walls of Jericho seven times. Also, Naaman dipped himself in the water seven times for healing." He went on and on about the number seven.

The doctor said, "You must be crazy."

"I am taking this news as a good sign," Dad said. "It's Not Over Until I Win!"

You Can't Keep a Good Man Down

My dad wanted to be back on a full travel schedule and my siblings and I were telling him, "You need to slow down and take care of yourself."

We even put him on restricted travel, but he kept sneaking out of the country for secret speaking engagements. I would find out on social media that he was in another country when people started posting pictures with him.

I would get so frustrated, because he had promised me, he was going to rest. I wanted to keep my father with me for as long as possible. I would call him, like I was the travel police and say, "Mr. Brown, when did you leave the States?"

He would say, "Oh, I just got a little off track. I'm so sorry. I'll be back shortly. I'm taking good care of myself, baby, I promise."

I would often exhaust myself trying to get him to slow down.

So, I decided to change my approach because I knew my father had no intention of taking it easy.

Therefore, I worked on managing the way that he travelled to ensure he did it wisely and arranged days for him to rest and restore.

I also made sure that when he got to his destination someone could bring healthy, organic or raw foods to the hotel, rather than him eating whatever was on the hotel menu or in the hotel room snack bar. I'd appoint someone, if I couldn't do it, to be the first to enter the room and remove temptations like candy or chips.

Important Healing Components

I genuinely believe that the holistic route we took, in addition to the traditional medicine we utilized, saved Dad's life. It made it possible for his body to heal itself, to the astonishment of the doctors. Even to this day, they are amazed by all that his body has endured and he is still out inspiring the world.

Now let's cover some of the specific steps we took that made a difference in him becoming a cancer conqueror.

Let's first emphasize my disclaimer: what I am sharing is based upon what we experienced in our journey to health. I am not a medical doctor and I can't say if the things I am going to talk about will work for you or not. Everyone's journey is different.

What I can highly recommend is that you do your own research, study and find out what works best for you, whether that be traditional medicine, holistic medicine, or a combination of both.

I am thankful for the doctors who care for my father. They are wonderful people with the heart to heal and want to do their best for their patients. Finding good, caring doctors may take a little time, but it is worth it. Don't ever be afraid to ask for a second or even third opinion. Take your health and the health of those you love seriously.

The Right Nutrients

Make sure that you are conscious of what you are putting into your body. You can't give the body death and expect to have life. Feeding life into the cells is so important and so crucial when you are in a place of healing.

You can't do the things that you used to do — you have to raise the bar for yourself, set a higher standard and be very selective about what you're putting into your body, because, when you are rising above a physical challenge, you're not living to eat .... you're eating to live.

Your Mindset

Having enough mental power not to accept whatever you've been told is crucial. If someone looks at you and says those three words no one wants to hear — You have _____ — it takes mental stamina to handle it and continue living each day to the fullest, no matter what. Maybe you are in the final chapter of your life, but you can be there on your own terms. You don't have to be depressed or sad. You can enjoy the time you have left.

I love, in the Bible, in the Book of Daniel, Chapter 3, where it talks of Shadrach, Meshach and Abednego. They told King Nebuchadnezzar, "Our God, whom we serve, is able to deliver us from the burning, fiery furnace and He will deliver us from your hand. But if not, let it be known to you, O king, that we will not bow . . . "

That's a similar space that we worked from to hold the vision. We didn't know if my father would make it or not, but we did everything we could to make sure he stayed on this side of life. I am so glad that we did. Every sacrifice was worth it.

Your Healing Space

Even though each component was vital to Dad's healing, there is one that is not talked about much, one that I believe strongly in and that is creating an environment that is conducive to healing.

Whether you are at home or in the hospital, create a peaceful place that calms the spirit. Every bit of stress robs an ounce of strength from the body. Utilize candles, incense, frankincense and/or essential oils, which are also a form of aromatherapy. Play music that calms the soul. Have pictures on the walls that induce peace and tranquility. Create your own place of restoration, which makes it easier to reflect and relax.

When people come into my space, they often say, "There is a very peaceful, very calming presence here." This is my prayer for anyone who enters my door:
"let them feel peace, let them feel that they have come out of the fast-paced, unpredictable twists and turns of the world and stepped into a haven where they can replenish, renew and recharge themselves."

Limiting Access

"My father said there were two kinds of people in the world: givers and takers. The takers may eat better, but the givers sleep better."
Marlo Thomas

When you are going through any type of major transition, it is important to surround yourself with givers. Keep a healthy space between you and the takers, because they will have a heyday. "Great—you're not using your car; let me borrow your car. You're not going anywhere; let me wear your shoes. Is there anything else I can take while you're out of commission?"

Because of this, I became the gatekeeper for my father. That was really challenging and I learned a lot about myself in the process.

"Adversity introduces a man to himself."
Albert Einstein

I am a person who likes to be liked and I love making people feel accepted and valued. So, learning to say no and to do it from a loving space was very hard. However, I teach other people why it is so important to set clear boundaries. You don't have to be mean, yet you do have to be firm. You can decline with love and remain focused on the main objective of healing yourself.

It doesn't mean I don't like you, it doesn't mean you're beneath me and it doesn't mean you are not important. It just means that, in this case, what is best for my father's healing is to use his energy, which is life force, wisely. You will not drain him in my presence.

When my dad was on his back, fighting for his life, some people still wanted to pull from him. "Can you help me get some speaking engagements?" "I need some money to cover my mortgage." One man he had been mentoring and helping called one of my father's clients, who had booked Dad for an engagement about nine months in advance and said, "You guys need to go ahead and book me instead, because Les isn't going to be here. The doctors have told him he is dying. You should go ahead and start advertising me as the keynote speaker, because he is not going to make it anyway." That was such a tough blow.

I started protecting Dad, screening all of his calls and making sure he was exposed to people for only a certain amount of time a day. The few people allowed to be around were made to understand that they had just a few moments and that they were not to request anything of him mentally, emotionally, spiritually, physically, or financially. Nothing was to be asked of him except that he get well.

I remember the great Jim Rohn called. He said, "Whatever he needs, if there is anything I can do, here's my home number, here's my cell number, here's my assistant's number. If it's financial, if it's mental, if it's emotional, whatever he needs, do not hesitate to call and ask. I am here. I love your father; he is like a brother to me. He is an amazing spirit and the world needs him to be here. You are not alone."

I just cried on the phone. First of all, I was so shocked. I had listened to Jim as I grew up and I met him backstage at an event where we had all spoken together in the New Orleans Superdome to 15,000 people. We were waiting backstage and I was shaking all over with fear that I would not be able to say one word in front of so many people. And Mr. Rohn told me, "You can do this, you've got this."

Dad had been saying the same thing to me, but when Jim said it, I thought, "Okay, maybe I can do this."

Mr. Jim said he had gone through a lot to get in contact with Dad because he wanted to hear my father's voice and know that he was alright. His sincere concern for my father was very heartwarming. I felt his love through the phone. He and Dad talked, they laughed, shared a couple of old stage stories, reflected a little bit and then Mr. Rohn started to speak life into him.

I could see it really touched my father and it was very healing for Mr. Rohn to reach out to him, brother to brother, speaker to speaker, to say "You matter. I care and I'm here for you in the midst of your troubles."

It Doesn't End

Once you are able to overcome a physical challenge, then the big problem becomes maintaining the healthy state. You can't treat healing, especially when you have something as serious as a cancer prognosis, like a simple cold.

We had many challenging conversations as a family, because in Dad's mind he was totally fine. He would say, "Everything is in remission, I'm doing good, I feel great. Can I just go ahead and do these fifteen engagements in two weeks? Eat what I want to eat and do what I want to do now?"

My answer would always be the same. "No, you cannot. We just had a miracle. We just came out of the dungeon of sickness, soaring high into health and wellness and you are ready to plunge us back into the pits of pain and disease? No. It doesn't mean that you act as if everything is okay."

Every day that my father is still here and is able to do what he loves to do is not taken lightly. I'm grateful, I'm appreciative and I am constantly reminding him that we are still in the process of defying the odds.

I tell him, "We cannot forget. We cannot allow our old behaviour patterns or our lack of discipline back in to your reality. We must commit to living a life of abundance. Let us not forget and fall prey to a life we don't want. Do you want to be bedridden again? Do you want to have to go through any type of radiation-seed treatment?"

"No, I don't."

"Okay, then let's move accordingly. Let's act accordingly. Let's make good choices."

I still have to be the gatekeeper and I still have to be the bad guy, or should I say bad girl, at times, but, so far . . . so good.

You have a divine appointment and your destiny is awaiting you. If you are struggling with your health, take a proactive approach. Be open to the possibilities and opportunities that may come your way. You gained access to this body of work for a reason. Continue to do your research and decide to live as long as you can and as big as you can. Just because a doctor recommends something doesn't mean that you have to do it. Find out what works for you and whatever you do, don't quit. Don't give up on your dreams.

We would love to stay connected with you. Visit Onabrown.com for all of your self-development and training needs. Also, let us know how you are owning your dreams.

13

In closing, be encouraged by the powerful words my father has been pouring into people around the world for years: No matter what you are facing, always remember, YOU HAVE GREATNESS within YOU. Say to yourself, It's Not Over Until I Win!

Growing in peace, love and gratitude,

Dr. Ona Love Brown
The Dream Queen and The Message Midwife!

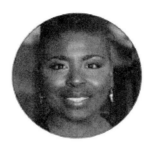

About
Dr. Ona Brown

Dr. Ona Brown has made her mark as an expert in personal and professional transformation throughout the world, inspiring and motivating audiences in hundreds of cities in the U.S. as well as numerous locations abroad including London, England; Sydney, Australia; Johannesburg, South Africa and Stockholm, Sweden.

She is also the "success-ologist" who escorts individuals, teams, corporations and non-profits on the journey to discovering how to excel beyond any seeming limitations and/or obstacles by activating their personal and professional power.

Ms. Brown has motivated tens of thousands throughout the United States and in over seven different foreign countries in the past 23 years. Ona Brown is a proven self-development vehicle, providing accelerated success strategies by awakening undiscovered personal power, boundlessly expanding visions and building sky-scraping dreams.

15

Chapter 2

My Journey to
Health, Wealth and Happiness

By: Mr. Raymond Harlall

My task in this chapter is to help you to transition from a difficult and unhealthy way of living to a truly purposeful life. The vast majority of people are victims of mental slavery. Specifically, your behaviour is a result of subliminal advertising, fulfilling the agenda and dreams of the super wealthy. How? Via billboards, radio and television advertisement to name the big ones. You fall into the trap set by mass media, leaving you wanting a celebrity-like lifestyle. In this chapter I hope to shed new light on how to take a more pivotal, positive and proactive approach to life—specifically as it pertains to your personal health, wealth and happiness.

Please do not be one of the masses of people, who live reactively, going with the flow, never planning for a rainy day. When life throws them a curveball, they miss, then blame everyone, but themselves for striking out. What do successful people do? They take a proactive approach to life. Successful people take responsibility for their actions, especially if that action resulted negatively.

This is where the magic happens. Healthy people live for the future, not the now. Wealthy people consider their health to be their most valuable asset, simply because wealth cannot buy health. The problem for centuries has been the middle class and poor are trying to get rich by trading hours for money. There are only 168 hours in each week. Therefore, working minimum wage will never make you rich no matter how many hours you work.

How then, are there so many self-made millionaires in the world today? They must have found a way to make money while they sleep. They have learned how to work once and keep getting paid; day in day out with positive cash flow, month after month. Wealthy people have learned how to create multiple streams of income. They have learned time is not only money, but more importantly, time is very precious. Time itself is an asset and it cannot be recovered once lost.

Fortunately, as you achieve more time and money, your only focus is your ability to stay healthy. The secret to maintaining this, is to achieve a work-life balance. The problem with this is only a small percent of the world's population is able to achieve financial freedom before they get old and even worst; stricken with ailments. I go into more details about money in my book ""The Handbook to Financial Freedom by 30"; A Millennial Guide to Rise Above the Rat Race!" Get your copy at RaymondHarlall.com

Now with all the cards are on the table, the challenge lies in the way you execute your master plan to achieve your dream life. The secret to being truly successful is to move from the low end of the spectrum to the high end gradually and continuously; to transcend from a state of obesity, poverty and stress; to obtain a physically fit body, multiple streams of residual income and exist in a space of total well-being.

To prove to you how backwards society has become. Let me ask you two questions? Do you go to the doctor to achieve optimum health or only when you are sick, if at all? How often do you take your car in to the dealer for 'preventative maintenance'?

After much research, I have concluded people take better care of their cars compare to their own health. On average North Americans will buy 12 cars in a life time. Can you believe we are all operating in a society such as this! Given the fact, our heart and body as a whole works 24 hours per day, 365 days a year multiplied by, eighty years on average. Therefore, it is necessary to pay keen attention to what you consume physically, mentally, spiritually and emotionally to keep our body, mind and spirit 100 percent functional.

Doctors Are Needed, But...

I googled 'Doctor Jokes' and found this one at www.workjoke.com and thought you might like it.

"A man speaks frantically into the phone,
"My wife is pregnant and her contractions are only two minutes apart!"
"Is this her first child?" the doctor queries.
"No, you idiot!" the man shouts. "This is her husband!"

Doctors and medicine are great, but only to identify and treat imminent or existing conditions. By most accounts, a doctor was the very first face you have seen on this earth, even before your own mother. However, the problem lies in their reactive practices in the treatment of symptoms as oppose to identifying and eliminating the root cause of the illnesses. Consuming routine prescription medication is not the way to live happy, healthy and wealthy.

Have you ever wondered why most prescription medications have a side effect? This is a systematic problem that runs deep into politics and is controlled by the super-rich and powerful. Thus, it is in your best interest to be educated.

7 Health Tips You Can Apply Right Now

Three of them are things to stop doing, the other 3 are recommendations to practice and the very last is about you realizing your greatness dwells within you.

1. Stop Being Proud of Your Diagnosis

Do not start the sentence with, "My doctor said I have..." People seem to be so proud of their diagnosis these days. It seems to give validation for them to continue with their routine of bad habits and they expect others to go easy on them. Yes, I understand it may be sad news initially, but do not entertain the idea of living with this condition. Read Ona Brown's chapter about Les Brown story of how he fought the 'Big C.'

2. Stop Seeking Pity for Your Current Medical Condition

If a car has a cracked windshield, do you feel sorry for the windshield, the car, or the owner—or would it be better to fix the windshield? You can heal yourself holistically. Read the other amazing chapters in this book and connect with the co-authors at h3book.com to help you create a health plan.

3. Stop Owning Your Medical Condition

Although we cannot trade our body in to the doctor for a new one like we can trade in our old vehicle, what is most important to understand is your body is always in equilibrium, the ultimate centre for disease control. We are only what we know we are! The old saying "Knowledge is power" is very true and extremely powerful if applied to the realms of health and wellness. Just be guarded with what you consume and consider hiring a Health and Wellness Coach. You will find several of them in this book.

4. Start Shifting Your Paradigm - Change Your Thinking Pattern

To be healthy, you must first think like the healthy version of yourself. January 1st of each year should not be the only day for you to set goals— most people never take action or continue for more than twenty-one days anyway. Why is this so hard? After all, a new year's resolution is a personal decision. Nine times out of ten the roadblock is in the execution of the goal. This is because the brain is the ultimate control centre and it governs itself. The brain creates and validates its own excuses as to why it's better to procrastinate, to wake up later, to eat fast food, to smoke, or to drink excessively or to do nothing at all.

5. Start Thinking Outside the Box - the Shortcut to Success

How do you achieve your dream life? The one-word answer is, mentorship. Find someone who's living the life you want and do what they do. Research them, get to know their story of struggle and their path to success. Read their books, watch their interviews and try to hire them as a coach. To watch interviews with me and my fellow co-authors, go to my YouTube channel Raymond & Friends TV.

6. Start Being Purposeful with the End Results in Your Mind

The definition of insanity is doing the same thing over and over again and expecting a different result. If left unchecked, you will be like a ship at sea without any map or sense of direction, just drifting in the wind. As the great Jim Rohn said, "It's not about the direction of the wind, but the set of your sail that will ultimately determine where you go." To get your mind to operate as if it's on a train track, with a set destination, you need to have a vision board.

7. Keep Swimming Against the Tide

Stop following the masses. As the famous one-liner said, "To go where you have never been, you need to do something you have never done." Be the change you want to see in the mirror. Learn to trust your instinct and make decisions that benefit you. Do more of what you are good at and delegate everything else, so you can get closer to your goals faster.

My mentor, Dr. George Grant and I, in collaboration with Les and Ona Brown and our fellow co-authors, coming under the umbrella of the *World Organization of Natural Medicine* ™, have decided to put this book together. Our goal, is to help you live a long, wonderful, healthy and purposeful life. Each co-author has shared his/her expertise and I am thankful.

I would love to connect with you and hear your story. Send an email to RaymondHarlall@icloud.com with your story of struggle and/or success and I will enter your name to win a signed copy of this book, mailed to your home.

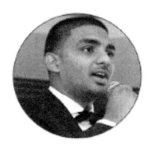

About
Mr. Raymond Harlall

Mr. Raymond Harlall owns several businesses and enjoys a six figure per year income doing what he loves. He is the author of three books, including co-authoring with New York Times best-selling author Dr. Brian Tracy. He is also the Award-Winning Author of "The Handbook to Financial Freedom by 30" foreword by New York Times best-selling author Mr. Raymond Aaron. He owns and operates a large transportation company; inclusive of a trucking company, an auto sale, a car-rental service, a taxi service and driving schools internationally.

Raymond is also a video-marketing coach, a motivational speaker, a philanthropist and a 'Youtuber' with over 1.3 million views with audiences in 224 countries. To watch over 100 of his Free Training Videos, visit his YouTube Channel by googling his name; 'Raymond Harlall'.

Raymond's passion, vision and mission; is to serve humanity and to give back by sharing his knowledge, skills and expertise. Specifically, he wants to share how you can stop working hard and start working smarter, so you can maintain perfect health, maximize wealth and ultimately, achieve peace of mind.

Chapter 3

26 Tips From A-Z to Live Healthy, Wealthy, Sexy and Wise to 101

By: Prof. Dr. George Grant
PhD, IMD, DHS

My family lived lives of quiet desperation while they suffered the effects of heart disease, diabetes and obesity. I watched my mother struggle with bypass surgery after bypass surgery only for her to die in her early forties from a heart attack. My father passed the same way twenty years later. It broke my heart and I knew I needed to do something about it.

I decided to dedicate my life to helping everyone live long and strong to age 101. I studied biochemistry, genetics, food science and nutrition, pharmacology and toxicology in my three undergraduate degrees and earned doctorate degrees in stress and integrative medicine with a focus on prevention instead of intervention. I followed this up later with a master's degree in food science and nutrition and became known as Dr. George the Caring Doctor.

Using my experience in integrative medicine and western allopathic medicine, I helped many of my clients recover fully from diabetes, hypertension, heart problems, fibromyalgia, MS, dementia, obesity and depression using natural methods along with their medical regimen until they experienced full recovery in four to six months. It is a joy to watch people recover their health and live their life to the fullest.

In this chapter, I am going to give you twenty-six tips to start you on this process to full health and longevity. Try acting on one tip a day and you will notice results as you continue putting my advice into action.

26 Tips From A-Z
Tip #1: Attitude
Have a positive mental attitude [PMA] no matter what. Having an attitude of gratitude will enhance your aptitude, which will form your altitude. Start and end your day with lots of PMA to lift your spirit and attract health, happiness and prosperity to thrive to 101.

Tip #2: Beliefs
If your belief system is you can live to 101 regardless of your genes, you will create habits for health and wealth to help you thrive and overcome any physical or financial challenge regardless of the nature of the economy or where you live. Your healthy body and mind will help you create sound habits to become healthy, wealthy, sexy and wise till 101 and beyond.

Tip #3: Commitments

Your daily commitment to the wellness IQ/GPS at www.academyofwellness.com will help you enhance your physical, mental and spiritual health to prevent disease and help you realize your full potential to live to 101.

Tip #4: Determinations

Once you determine to change your daily healthy habits by increasing your consumption of raw or steamed organic vegetables, fruits, whole grains and nuts while reducing or eliminating your consumption of flour, sugar, sodas, coffee, processed foods and alcohol you will feel increased energy and vitality. Ensuring full hydration by drinking eight glasses of water with lemon, achieving an alkaline pH of 7.4 and practising deep breathing will help you achieve better physical and mental health till 101.

Tip #5: Enthusiasm

From the Latin *en Theos* (within God), this is an essential life skill for you to thrive physically, mentally and spiritually, which will attract wealth and other enthusiastic people to propel you forward to success in all areas of your life till 101.

Tip #6: Fun

Add daily, weekly and monthly fun in your life. Do what you love and love what you do to add more enjoyment in your life. Daily laughter is essential for optimal health. Let your smile change the world and never let the world change your smile. Taking regular vacations plays an essential part in adding fun and neutralizes excess stress so you can live happily to 101.

Tip #7: Gambling No More

You *cannot* afford to gamble with your health or wealth if you truly plan to live to 101. This is wellness by choice, not by chance. Understanding probability will save you thousands of dollars in buying lottery tickets or gambling in casinos, where the house must win to stay in business. Saving and investing regularly to stay debt free is much wiser than gambling and risking the capital you worked so hard to accumulate.

Tip #8: Happiness

Happy people always have a positive mental attitude and their enthusiasm is infectious. Try to be around happy people to lift your spirit and help you thrive to 101 instead of associating with negative people who pull you down and have a negative impact on your health and wealth. It is wise to be selective in choosing family and friends.

Tip #9: Investing

Investing in your health and wealth is an essential skill in living to 101. Regular exercise and minimizing stress, which contributes to 85 percent of all diseases, is an excellent investment in your health. Regular savings and wise investing are essential for financial wellness. Earning residual income or dividend income from safe stocks is better than depending on linear income. Have 5 percent of all your assets in gold and silver to protect you against inflation until 101.

Tip #10: Job

Your job and career can help you achieve total wealth and health if there is enjoyment and congruence between your personality and your career. If you are in a dead-end job or feel underemployed, it will have a negative impact on your health and wealth. Choosing your job and career wisely is an essential skill for you to live to 101.

Tip #11: Kindness

A daily habit of performing a random act of kindness will enhance your life. In fact, you are creating your destiny, even as you read this. That means . . . what you think of this very moment and the choices you make now, create the foundation of what you think is the future.

Once you understand this truth and experience its effects for yourself, you'll begin to understand first-hand you are the creator and master of your destiny.

You can then begin making sound choices for your inner well-being but for your outer circumstances by choosing random acts of kindness to 101.

Tip #12: Love

Showing unconditional love to God, family, friends, coworkers and associates creates balance and harmony in your life. Balancing physically, mentally and spiritually will help you achieve total wellness to 101.

Tip #13: Money

Your relationship to money will determine your wealth to 101. Money is an essential tool for survival, but the love of and lust for money is the root of all evil. You can trace wars, divorce, firings from jobs and any dispute back to greed and lust for money. Being content with what you have is critical for you to live healthy, wealthy and wise to 101.

Tip #14: Negating Negativity

Quieting the negative thoughts that spin you deeper and deeper into uncertainty about life is important for you to live a balanced life. Transforming whatever makes you unhappy into true spiritual abundance is an important life skill. Allow fears, doubts and worries to evaporate into unending quiet and peace of mind. Let the past be the past, a peaceful picture in your mind that has no grip on your presence in this moment. Remember, the past is history, the future is a mystery and today is the present. Enjoy it. Open yourself, moment by moment, to a solid sense of assurance, strength, balance and wisdom to thrive to 101.

Tip #15: Overachievement Avoidance

Do not confuse productivity with overachieving. Many overachievers suffer from stress and burnout. If you want to live to 101 and beyond, pace yourself. You have plenty of time to achieve all your goals and dreams without excess stress or burnout.

Tip #16: Prostrate Health

Since 50 percent of men over 50, 60 percent over 60, 70 percent over 70, 80 percent over 80, 90 percent over 90 and 100 percent over 100 suffer from an enlarged prostate, which may lead to prostate cancer and erectile dysfunction, it is imperative to keep your prostate healthy to enjoy sex after 100! As I am writing this book, I am doing research on a natural supplement to prevent and reverse an enlarged prostate. The research will be complete in six months and published in scientific journals.

Tip #17: Quiet Mind

Daily meditation and attaining a quiet mind by deep breathing and walking on the beach or in the woods, listening to the natural sounds of waves or birds will achieve quantum healing and help you reach 101.

Tip #18: Rest

Taking daily and frequent rest breaks are essential to rejuvenate your mind and reduce your stress. Resting the body and mind is a prerequisite in achieving total balance and wellness to 101.

Tip #19: Sex

This is not just for honeymooners or procreation, but should be enjoyed at any age as long as you are in perfect health. Most women during Men-a-Pause lose their libido and most men during andropause experience erectile dysfunction and lack of interest in intimacy. I recommend reading the book *Hot Women, Cool Solution* by Pat Duckworth (*Available on Amazon*).

Tip #20: Trust

Do you trust God, yourself, your loved one, your boss, your friends, your associates, your employees, or do you always live in a state of doubt? Achieving total balance requires total trust to live to 101.

Tip #21: Uterus Health

Many women suffer from uterine fibroids and ovarian cysts [PCOS] after menopause, which requires medication or surgery and can lead to complications. Good uterine health can be attained naturally by reducing consumption of sugar, animal products including dairy and fried and processed foods, as well as limiting alcohol consumption. Maintaining a healthy uterus is as important for women as maintaining a healthy prostate is for men to live healthy and sexy to 101.

Tip #22: Vacations

Taking regular vacations is a necessity, not a luxury, to maintain healthy balance in your life. I am fortunate to be able to take a working vacation every two months and I strongly recommend trying it at least twice a year. Taking a cruise or travelling to warm places during cold winter months is recommended to live to 101.

Tip #23: Weight Management

Maintaining a healthy weight or a healthy BMI (Body Mass Index) is critical to avoiding and reversing diabetes, hypertension, stroke and many other diseases that shorten your lifespan. Eat breakfast like a king/queen, lunch like a prince/princess and supper like a pauper to avoid obesity.

Tip #24: Youth

Can we feel youthful at 101? Yes, absolutely. If you follow the first twenty-three tips, you will be on your way to feeling healthy, wealthy, sexy, youthful and wise at 101 and beyond.

Tip #25: Zeal

This is the last foundation tip, which is probably the most important. Your zeal and eagerness to live to 101 will propel you on your pursuit of healthy living, sharpening your mind and exploring your full potential to help yourself and others on this wonderful journey.

Tip #26: Read and Practice the First Twenty-five Tips Daily for Twenty-six Days to Live and Thrive to 101+

Living healthy is not as hard as people think. Small changes over time can create big results. If you need help with your health, I am here for you. I am an active member of five professional organizations. I worked with ten Olympic athletes from Canada and the USA and three Nobel prize winners. I participated in conferences with Harvard, Mayo Clinic, Cleveland Clinic and Johns Hopkins.

I work part-time at my private integrative clinic in North York, Ontario and I work as a professor at WONM (World Organization of Natural Medicine), helping my students completing their training on biofeedback, orthomolecular nutrition, stress management and bio cranial therapy.

My goal is to inspire and empower clients, corporations and non-profits to live healthy to 101+ until I expire. My clients call me the Caring Doctor, since we care, serve and educate—not medicate, operate, irradiate, vaccinate or irritate.

Please feel free to check me out at www.DrGeorgeGrant.com and then book a time to talk. Let's see what we can do together to improve your health and help you to live to 101!

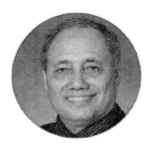

About
Prof. Dr. George Grant, PhD, IMD, DHS

Prof. Dr. George Grant, PhD, IMD., DHS., is known as The Miracle & Caring Doctor, is considered the Canadian authority in Integrative Medicine [IM] & Functional Medicine [FM] and Canada's Wellness Ambassador.

He pioneered the research on Beta Endorphins; organized and presented at the International Pain Conference in Chicago, IL; has helped several fortune 500 companies worldwide; non-profit organizations; and top Olympic Athletes.

Prof. Dr. Grant is an Editor of several refereed scientific journals, 270 published articles, 150 conference presentations, 280 book/paper reviews and 10 bestselling books.

Chapter 4

How to Overcome Midlife Crisis

By: Ms. Cora Cristobal

"What am I doing? Where am I going? What more is left in life?"

These were questions reverberating in my mind as I stood facing Lake Ontario.

Here I was, half a century old after a divorce, one problem teenage daughter, three other teenage children, a complete hysterectomy, a series of eye infections and an almost fatal car accident.

I was on my own as a sole parent in a new country, an immigrant in Canada from the Philippines. I never thought it was midlife crisis. All I knew was it was tough and I was in crisis . . .

It Was Time for A Change

That was when I started to look at life at a different level and with a different perspective.

At the lowest moment, I had only two choices: to stay miserable and just coast along, or to do something really special for a more meaningful life. I found myself spending more time alone, analyzing things, listening to the word of God. What is the lesson; what is the message . . .

"What am I doing? Where am I going? What more is left in life?"

Then I found myself visiting conservation parks, lakes, rivers and mountains, communing with nature. I enjoyed the solitude and I learned to meditate and pray in nature. As I did, God started to heal my heart as I cried out to Him. It helped me to have peace of mind.

I also started back on my reading and a motivational book inspired me to travel. As if by a miracle, I got a bonus from my employer which allowed me to travel to central Europe. I went to London, Paris, Switzerland and Italy. I was amazed by the grandeur and magnificent beauty of the many places I visited and the exquisite experience. At my last stop at the Basilica in Rome, I felt the Holy Spirit touch me and sweep away all my heartaches and pains as I cried with gratitude and joy. On the plane back to Toronto, I felt I was ready for a new life and there the old bubbly, energetic and happy Cora was back!

Not only did I work on the mental, spiritual and emotional side of myself, I also worked on my finances. In the Philippines, I had been a successful real estate broker. I decided to get my licence in Canada and started making extra money, which alleviated some of the stress.

The healing did not occur overnight. It took a couple of years for this whole process to happen. I learned it takes time and there are layers to the journey. Every time I let go, healing would come and I was able to move forward more. There came a point where I started to make leaps.

At the beginning, real estate only meant survival—a way of earning extra income. I still maintained my full-time job as a CPA (certified public accountant) with $35,000 in gross income. I did so well in my first six months with the real estate brokerage that my partner encouraged me to quit my job and I did. It was time for a change, but . . .

My previous employer maintained me as a consultant and paid me more money. They liked me and the work I did. I was able to do the job of two people because I was fast and efficient. I had also streamlined the processes in their accounts payable department.

In 2008 - 2009, Canada experienced a short recession in real estate and there was a lot of talk that Canada would follow the recession of the US. My employer fired the man who had replaced me because he could not perform and offered me my full-time job back at a higher pay with improved benefits. Who could turn that down? So, I went back, but I became very bored. Was it a symptom of a midlife crisis?

In 2015, I was ready for a change and I needed help to determine my next path, so I hired a mentor. It was one of the best decisions of my life. One of the things he suggested was writing a book, something to encourage others. So, I did it, in six weeks! No one had told me it should take longer and I was hungry to start the new stage of my life.

Things exploded afterwards. I got to share the stage with Jack Canfield, Brian Tracy and Robert Allen. I co-authored a book with celebrities and stars like Dr. John Gray, Marci Shimoff, Raymond Aaron, Sunil Tulsiani and Brian Tracy. It was an investment, but it was time for me to become who I was meant to be. I found ways and did whatever it took to make the extra money needed and my life was completely changed.

I also founded the Toronto Woman's Club - TorontoWomensClub.com, a hub where women (as well as men) can come, learn and grow into the people they were meant to be. It is my passion to help others and now I get to live the way I want, continuing with real estate full-time and committed to educate, inspire and empower men and women.

I continued my travels, going to western Europe and Spain as well as retreats in the Caribbean. And the doors opened to international speaking opportunities in the UK, USA and South Africa.

Midlife Crisis

I believe most people go through some sort of midlife crisis. For most people, it is not severe and it comes on as we age and start to reflect on our life. We look at what we have done and the things we still want to do and consider if they are possible. The crisis comes when we think we can't do it, that we are trapped forever in an unfulfilled life.

You see this especially in women who have focused for the last twenty to thirty years on raising a family. When the children are gone, they feel like they don't have any choices.

The other time you see it coming happening is with traumatic experiences, such as separation, divorce, or death.

What Are the Symptoms of Midlife Crisis?

The first one is spending more time alone. You don't want to talk to anyone. You feel isolated and like no one has been through or understands what you are going through. You don't want to deal with life anymore.

Number two is a deep sense of regret or remorse for goals not accomplished. You are already forty or fifty years old and you haven't done what you would have liked to do.

Three is feeling you are left behind. There is a sense of humiliation, because other people you know around your age are more successful.

Fourth is being obsessed with your appearance. I saw every grey hair and I had gained weight. As you get older, your metabolism slows down, especially in women reaching menopause. Every little thing I felt was wrong with me bothered me.

One thing to note, when women go into menopause, it changes moods and eating and sleeping habits. This can also trigger an onset of a midlife crisis.

Fifth is depression and suicidal thoughts. I see people in a midlife crisis with depression. They become miserable or sad. They cannot explain what it is. I am not a doctor or a psychologist; I am only talking from my own experience. There was one point where I seriously considered throwing myself into Lake Ontario and ending it all. I have clients who are in their late forties and early fifties who are going through depression; they go to doctors and they can't find anything wrong with them. In these cases, it could be a symptom of a midlife crisis.

Sixth is restlessness and starting to think about changing careers. You assess where you are. You are not happy with it and wonder if there is more. I completely changed my career. I had been a CPA for over twenty-five years and I could do my job with my eyes closed. Then I went into book writing, speaking and mentoring and it is new and exciting. I have come alive again.

Sometimes, when we are young, we end in up jobs we never liked, but we got trapped because they paid the bills. Then you hit midlife and you realize you can't take it anymore. The crisis hits because, even though you hate your job, you are secure in it. In my case, I had not wanted to become an accountant. It was not my dream.

Sometimes finding your purpose, your passion and your meaning happens during midlife. It's a symptom of a midlife crisis when you are tempted to change your career. What is it you would like to do?

Another symptom is boredom. When you get bored with what you normally do, it is an opportunity to look for a change in your career or to do something you want to do, especially when the kids are grown and no longer need you like they used to.

How to Conquer Midlife Crisis

I am not a doctor or a health professional, so what I am sharing here is what has helped me overcome my midlife crisis. If you feel it's beyond your ability to handle, then you need to seek professional help.

The one step that helped me greatly was to travel as much as possible. It opened up my mind to new things and the rest I got during my vacations helped me to think better when I was home.

Number two, I committed to regular exercise. I signed up for a gym membership in the community centre and I go there three to five times a week. This is good for my physical and mental well-being. It's not only about losing weight, but being healthy as well.

Number three, I would wake up at 5 in the morning and go for a walk in the park close to my house, where I would meditate. When I got home, I'd do more meditation and then journal about all the things I was thankful for. I also thought about and planned my day and set out my intentions. This helped me fill my day with productivity and success and not get overwhelmed.

We tend to work, work, work, but I think as we grow older and especially in our midlife, we need to spend more time thinking and making the decisions for our life.

Fourth, I got to know new people. I joined different entrepreneurial groups, where my mind was expanded to new possibilities in life. I learned new skills and hung around people who encouraged me to become the best me I could.

I changed my career. I started doing real estate on the side to earn extra money and it became my passion. What can you start to do that you love? Maybe it will lead to a new career or even just a hobby which inspires you and refreshes your soul. This is a great time to do something new in your life and discover your passions.

Fifth, I added more positivity to my life. I found things to make me laugh. I spent less time with people who dragged me down. I found things to inspire me and did those. You can too. What inspires you? Who are the people who lift you up? Hang around with those people. I also choose to look at life differently, to see the positive and not focus on the negative.

Sixth, I took my spirituality seriously. I learned how to have a deeper relationship with God and trust that He holds my life in His hands and this is a good place to be. Maybe you don't believe in God. If you don't, then I

41

encourage you to explore the possibility. Maybe you are unhappy because the spiritual side of you is crying out for more
.

You Can Survive It

I am living proof you can make it through a midlife crisis and come through it better than you were. The choice is yours. You can stay where you are miserable, or you can look at this as a new stage of your life where you can make a new start and become the person you were meant to be.

Recognize this is going to take time. It is going to take effort. Change does not happen easily and you will have to be prepared for the fact there will be bumps along the way.

But . . .

It is worth it. Don't live your life in regret, in the could-haves and should-haves. Live your life to the fullest, knowing you have done everything you have set out to do. The choice is yours.

Take a moment to stop and be still. Pause in silence and ask yourself:

- "Where am I going? What am I doing? What more is left in life?"
- "What am I called for to do for the remainder of my life?
- "If not now, when?"

Be sure to read Hailey's chapter if you are going through a tough time as a teenager or a young lady.

I would love to connect with you. I also would love to gift you with a copy of any of my books. Please contact me at cora@torontowomensclub.com.

To a fulfilled life,
Cora

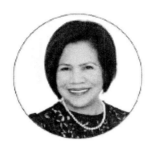

About
Ms. Cora Christobal

Ms. Cora Christobal is the founder of the Toronto Women's Club (TWC), Award Winning and International Best-Selling Author, Mentor, International Speaker, Real Estate Investor / Realtor / Consultant. A CPA by profession, Cora was a successful accounting professional having worked with multinational companies then embarked on a highly rewarding real estate career.

She has co-authored books with Dr. John Gray, Marci Shimoff, Raymond Aaron, Brian Tracy. She has shared stages with legends Jack Canfield, Brian Tracy and Robert Allen speaking about transformation, personal growth and acquiring wealth through real estate. Cora is an avid international traveler and enjoys making new friends, connections and collaborations. She is producing a big event in Toronto on April 6, 2019, which is bringing Jack Canfield, the co-author of the phenomenal "Chicken Soup For The Soul" and "The Secret"

.

Chapter 5

Oral Health and Systemic Health

By: Dame Dr. Sheila McKenzie,
RDH, PhD, DHMS, DHS

A Self-Care-in-Action Approach

The information contained in this chapter is based on research, my education and my personal and clinical experience. It is not intended as a substitute for consultation with your healthcare provider. For treatment and diagnosis of disease conditions or for drug therapy, please visit a healthcare provider.

My experience in oral systemic integration started over thirty years ago. As a trained dental professional, I tried to deliver the best level of dental care in accordance with my education. But often clients would return with the same bleeding gums, mouth ulcers, receding gum margins, sensitive teeth and many other signs of systemic health issues were evident in the mouth. I decided I must find a more integrative approach to help the patients who failed to respond to standard care.

During my research, I came across a magazine at a health-food store and read an article on orthomolecular nutrition subclinical signs of vitamin C. I was intrigued by the article and understood then that some of my clients' symptoms were related to subclinical manifestation of scurvy. I came to an understanding, as a healthcare provider, my training did not prepare me for a more integrative approach to healing.

I embarked on a journey of learning more about healing. I was on a mission and pursued avenues of learning as I could. I attended seminars, workshops and conferences; took university postgraduate courses; and completed a degree in orthomolecular nutrition at a time when it was not as popular as it is now. I was fortunate to attend Dr. Linus Pauling's lectures on more than one occasion.

In addition to studying orthomolecular nutrition, I obtained a doctorate in homeopathic medicine. In my estimation, I have attended more than 500 workshops, seminars, lectures and conferences on integrative medicine, orthomolecular nutrition, homeopathy and dental medicine. Manual techniques and other holistic healing techniques, I also lecture to many groups, professional organizations, gust on TV and radio, wrote articles for various magazines including the Lifestyle and Wellness magazine which I was the editor of for over ten years. My mission is to get the message to as many individuals as I can on the importance of the mouth and the systemic health,

In the early days of introducing the concept in my practice, I was so excited. I had vitality not only in my body, but my mind and began to slowly introduce orthomolecular nutrition and homeopathic immune system support into my practice. However, my dental colleagues and a medical physician in the clinic where I worked were outright sceptical and rude about my approach.

What was really puzzling to me was the failure of the clinicians to see the relationship between nutrition and clients' health challenges. I remember the only nutrition advice one of the dentists would suggest to clients was not to consume sugary foods between meals, but instead to consume it with the main meal. The reasoning was the sugar would have less contact with the teeth during the main meal. I suggested patients should receive probiotics after being prescribed antibiotics and he laughed at me. I knew then I was working with an ignorant group of clinicians who were not only in the dark ages, but were unwilling to move toward the light.

I decided to open a private orthomolecular nutrition-counselling practice while I continued in the dental practice. I would encourage receptive clients to schedule appointments for orthomolecular nutritional guidance and homeopathic immune stem supportive care. Over the years, I grew my practice into a fully integrative health service with special emphasis on periodontal health and the relationship between systemic, chronic pain syndromes and immune health challenges. Due to the space limitations of this chapter I will focus on periodontal health.

It has been my experience many people like to get to "the diagnosis" so they can get to the "treatment." I also feel unsettled when clients make statements like "I am here for you to fix me, doc. I've gone to many doctors already, but I am still sick." To which, I would reply, "What are you willing to do?"

At the first complimentary consultation, which I offer to all potential clients, I clarify the philosophy of natural integrative medicine. It is not about focusing on the disease label, but on the person with the disease.

Just before writing this chapter I read a Facebook post in which the participant stated, "I'm so tired of pain, loneliness, crying, guilt, struggling daily to take all those medications, missing out on life because of my fibromyalgia." Notice how the poster claimed the title of the disease: "my fibromyalgia."

I responded she had a choice. I also wondered why, in these days of information overload, people were still stumbling in the dark. I posted a link to my Self-Care in Action© link on my website, www.drsheilamckenzie.com. I am still waiting to see if she will act.

The techniques and suggestions I offer my clients and the basic version offered in this book are applicable to multiple, if not all, health challenges. In general terms, it's about decreasing oral and systemic inflammation with orthomolecular nutrition techniques and homeopathic immune system support. If you live, breathe, or know someone who ever gets sick, then the suggestions in this book are pertinent to you.

The public at large are accustomed to visiting various healthcare providers for different areas of the body. For example, a few years ago I was invited to participate in a radio show. The interviewer asked me about my profession and when I told him the focus of my practice was oral health and homeopathy, he responded oral medicine was medicine taken by mouth and homeopathy was medicine taken at home. I was totally flabbergasted, but kept my composure and stuck to polite answers.

Oral health means the health of the mouth. The oral medicine branch of medicine focuses on the mouth is known in dentistry as stomatology: dentistry concerned with the structures, functions and diseases of the mouth.

Homeopathy is a holistic system of medicine based on the principle of "like cures like" - that is, a substance which can cause symptoms when taken in large doses, can be used in small amounts to treat similar symptoms. The aim is creating an immune response and start the body's own healing mechanisms. The basic concept of allopathic (modern medical drug system of medicine) vaccination was borrowed from the philosophy of homeopathy.

The basic techniques of how it is practiced was established over 200 years ago by a German physician, Samuel Hahnemann, who was looking for a way to reduce the damaging side effects associated with the allopathic medical treatment of his day. The principle of treating "like with like" dates to Hippocrates (460 – 377 BC). There are basically two forms of practicing homeopathy, the classical, this style of homeopathy is very comprehensive and is practiced by well trained homeopaths while, contemporary homeopathy is less complicated and use more combination treatment and remedies. As a trained homeopath (doctor of homeopathy level of education) I incorporate homeopathic medicine according to the specific needs of the clients. However, there are some basic homeopathic, remedies and minerals that can be safely used for self-care which I will recommend later.

I also asked a family member who is an allopathic physician what her understanding was of the profession of dental hygienist. Her answer was they clean teeth. This indicates a significant lack of understanding from other healthcare providers and the public at large, about this important aspect of healthcare.

For clarification, a Registered Dental Hygienist (RDH) is a primary healthcare provider who is trained in detecting and initiating treatment for health issues of the oral cavity, including cancer screening and checking for nutritional deficiencies. Many diseases, because they are first evidenced in the mouth, are detected by dentists and dental hygienists before they are noted by other healthcare providers.

Preventive dental healthcare starts at the time of pregnancy, but due to the limitation of this chapter, I cannot dive more deeply into the subject.

You will not have good general health if you don't have good oral health. "The mouth is part of the body" is now considered an obvious statement. Oral diseases are most often indications of systemic diseases. Over the years, I have detected many systemic health challenges, to name a few such as colitis, vitamin B12 deficiency, anaemia digestive disorders, candidiasis, blood sugar imbalance and other conditions too numerous to include here. By examining the mouth, analyze and provide effective integrative interventions to correct such imbalances. In fact, I teach tongue diagnostic technique to healthcare professionals. To approach oral dental health by simply dealing with the immediate vicinity of the problem area in the mouth is like walking on one leg. With the one-leg approach, you are never totally balanced.

It has been estimated more than 100 systemic diseases and upward of 500 conditions have oral manifestations, which are typically more prevalent in the older population. (Journal of General Dentistry, November 2017.) Hippocrates reportedly cured systemic conditions by pulling infected teeth. Despite this, the relationship and impact of oral conditions on systemic conditions have not been fully appreciated until recently. It is now supported by scientific evidence. It took lengthy scientific research to conclude what has been known since 370 BC, even though most dental and medical providers are still offering the one-leg approach.

What Is Periodontal Disease?

The term "periodontal disease" is used to describe a group of conditions causing inflammation and destruction of the attachment apparatus of the teeth (i.e., gingiva, periodontal ligament, root and jaw bone). According to the standard dental text, periodontal disease is caused by bacteria found in dental plaque (a film of slime that adheres to tooth surfaces).

While the condition usually starts as a simple gum irritation, if untreated, it can become a full-blown disease. Periodontal disease is the major cause of tooth loss in people, even as young as thirty-five. More than 50 percent of the population has at least the early stages of gingivitis. Three out of four adults are eventually affected by periodontal disease. Many natural healthcare systems recognize periodontal disease may be a sign of deeper trouble in the immune system.

What Are the Basic Signs of Gum Disease?

Gums that bleed when you brush your teeth; red, swollen or tender gums; gums that have receded or shrunk away from your teeth indicate gum disease. In advanced cases there can be pus between the teeth and gums when the gums are pressed; teeth that loosen or change position, often causing the front teeth to fan out; a change in one's bite; a change in the way a partial denture fits; bad breath or a chronic bad taste in one's mouth; along with teeth sensitivity. According to orthodox dentistry, it is related to "the germ theory," or "the bacteria".

1. Theory of Bacterial Plaque

According to conventional dental textbooks, bacterial plaque (a soft, sticky transparent film that adheres to the teeth) is the causative agent in most forms of periodontal disease. Bacteria are known to produce and secrete numerous toxins detrimental to the health of the tissues.

In my opinion and many other holistic minded healthcare professionals for the gums to be healthy, the rest of the body, including normal protective elements that help the body guard against diseases, must also be healthy. The fact is, all humans and other living creatures as well, harbour millions of bacteria in their mouth and other body cavities. Most of the time, they cause no harm. They are, in fact, a necessary part of our body's ecosystem.

We have all seen commercials selling products that claim to kill nasty bad breath, help prevent gum disease, or ward off tooth-decay germs; however, we continue to wage a fruitless war against bacteria. We must begin strengthening our body's natural bacterial-control mechanisms. Periodontal disease is caused by many things which disturb the bacterial colonies in the mouth or upset the normal biochemical balance of the whole body.

2. Tartar and Periodontal Disease

Another cause of periodontal disease, according to the many orthodox dental textbooks I have studied, is tartar (a hardened mineral deposit on the teeth that cannot be removed by normal brushing) is the problem. But I often wonder what comes first: the chicken or the egg? Tartar has a rough surface which irritates the gum tissue and provides a site for the accumulation of plaque. Is tartar calcified plaque or not?

To answer this question, let's examine the components of tartar. It is a mineralized mass with various minerals, such as you would normally find in bone — namely calcium, calcium carbonate, calcium phosphate, magnesium, etc. There are also trace minerals in it such as iron, zinc, copper and fluoride (it is interesting to note the amount of fluoride in tartar is influenced by the amount of fluoride in the drinking water, topical application and dentifrices.

Several stages, according to the textbooks, occur from bacterial plaque to tartar, but is it the bacteria or an imbalance in the body that causes extensive precipitation of minerals in the saliva? The body fluids of healthy individuals are alkaline (have a high pH), whereas the body fluids of unhealthy individuals are acidic (have a low pH). Many degenerative diseases, including periodontal disease, have been linked to mineral deficiencies (especially ionic calcium).

Many people come to my clinic every three months to have tartar removed from their teeth. Despite this, some of these regular patients appear as if their teeth haven't been cleaned in years, while those who have in fact not had their teeth cleaned in years appear to have had their teeth cleaned recently. Many of those with excessive tartar are not any less diligent in their oral hygiene habits.

It is beyond the scope of this book to go into more depth as to the formation of tartar, but it is sufficient to know that tartar, regardless of how it gets on your teeth, should be removed to maintain the health of the gum tissue. When patients have a constantly heavy buildup of tartar on their teeth, a mineral screening and minerals balancing is called for, which I include for all clients.

3. Restorations and Periodontal Disease

Faulty fillings are common causes of irritation and destruction of the periodontal tissues. If margins of fillings are not smooth and contoured to the teeth, an ideal site will be formed for the accumulation of plaque and irritation of the surrounding tissues by bacterial toxins. If the restoration is of silver amalgam, there might be more periodontal involvement due to the decreased activities of antioxidant enzymes.

Mercury accumulation results in a depletion of free-radical scavenging enzymes (such as glutathione peroxide, Sulfur oxide dismutase and catalase). The connective tissue is particularly sensitive to free radical damage. If you notice a bluish or black stain in the gumline and on the side of your tongue next to an amalgam filling (filling with a combination of mercury and other metals), it is a sign that the filling is deteriorating and spilling its mercury content into the surrounding tissues. It is wise to get it removed, but remember, before any filling with mercury is removed, a chelation detoxification therapy must commence for at least two weeks before and continue for up to four weeks after. Chelation therapy is done in my practice to remove toxic elements, reducing systemic inflammation and supporting the immune system.

From time to time, many individuals ask my opinion on the safety of silver amalgam fillings. Well, I will reserve my opinions, but the World Health Organization advises there are no safe levels of mercury.

Drugs and Periodontal Disease

Drugs can lower the resistance of the tissues to periodontal disease (e.g., steroids suppress the immune system)

Hormonal Changes

Hormonal fluctuation such as prepuberty, pregnancy or menopause, can also alter the defense mechanism of the body and contribute to periodontal disease

Miscellaneous Causes

Chemical irritants, such as those in cigarettes, lower the amount of oxygen in the blood steam, increase the need for antioxidants and impede the body's ability to heal itself.

Genetics and Susceptibility to Periodontitis

Vulnerability to periodontitis depends on each person's immune response. These are noted to have contributed to the likelihood of aggressive periodontitis; defects of the tissues that line the body surface (epithelial tissue), tissues that connect, support and separate other tissues (connective tissues) and the cells that produce collagen in the connective tissues (fibroblasts). For more information on genetics and periodontal disease see references.

Nutritional Deficiencies and Compromised Immunity

According to holistic views of disease, which I completely agree with, is that it is not as an enemy, one does not get attacked by microbes and fungi, but as a manifestation of the breakdown of the mechanisms that maintain control, resistance and balance.

Two-time Nobel prize winner Dr. Linus Pauling declared "nearly all disease can be traced to a nutritional deficiency." Vitamin C deficiency is associated with defective formation of the connective tissues that hold cells together (collagen), delayed healing of tissues and poor bone calcification. If your vitamin C levels drop too low, you could develop scurvy; in fact, bleeding gums is one of the first signs of scurvy. In addition to vitamin C, other signs of vitamin deficiencies such as Vitamin B12, is associated with bleeding and swollen gums, vitamin A is essential for collagen synthesis as well as healing of tissues and enhancing many immune functions throughout the body.

It is now supported by scientific research that dysbiosis of the oral microbiota can interfere with the normal function of the host immune system, resulting in enhanced development of periodontitis. Problems show up all over your body when your intestinal bacteria are imbalanced. Often, the signs can be seen in your mouth. Your oral microbiome and gut microbiome are co-dependent. Dysbiosis of Salivary Microbiota in Inflammatory Bowel Disease and Its Association with Oral Immunological Biomarkers - DNA Research, Volume 21, Issue 1, 1 February 2014, Pages 15 - 25.

Orthodox Periodontal Disease Diagnosis

The standard, conventional approach to diagnosing periodontal disease is to measure tooth mobility, check bleeding points in your gums (bleeding index) and measure pocket depth—the space between the teeth and the gum tissue—with a special instrument known as a periodontal probe. The extent of the gum disease is determined by the "pocket measurement," clinical examination and x-rays determine the extent of the gum disease.

In my practice in addition to the standard approach, the integrative examination consists of whole-body, two-segment examination, namely the external and the internal. The external examination consists of reading blood pressure, observing breathing, taking an energy index and head and neck palpation of lymph nodes. Thermography may be included to help assess inflammation, which may be present in the head region, along with mineral screening to determine nutritional status, endocrine balance and oral nitric oxide test as inflammatory marker.

Nitric Oxide Check for Inflammatory Markers

Nitric oxide synthases (NOS) are a family of isoforms (one of several different structurally similar proteins responsible for the synthesis of the potent dilator **nitric oxide** (NO). Expression of **inducible**NOS (iNOS) occurs in conditions of inflammation and produces large amounts of NO. Nitric oxide synthesis is increased in inflamed periodontal tissues. Also, studies have shown increased salivary concentrations of nitric oxide in patients with periodontitis. I include Nitric oxide as part of my assessment technique in my practice.

Sometimes clients ask why I use thermography for this reason I include dental practice. Dental health is linked to overall health; many dental health issues can be linked to other general health issues like headaches, neck pain and sinus inflammation. Thermography makes it possible to monitor the heat patterns from the mouth that run to other parts of the body like the thyroid and breasts. It is part of the assessment technique in my integrative assessment approach.

Signs of systemic diseases, such as diabetes and cancer, as well as other concerns like candida and vitamin and mineral deficiencies can be detected by your dental professional before your medical doctor is aware of them. After examining all the areas of your mouth, a soft-tissue exam is done—examination of your tongue, throat, colour of tissues, saliva consistency, your teeth and supporting structures position of your teeth cavities, etc.

Minimum-dose x-rays can be used in dental practice to identify cavities that cannot be detected by observation and bone loss. Loosing bone in the jaw is a sign of loosing bone elsewhere in the body: osteoporosis. Bad breath and bleeding gums could be indicators of diabetes. A sore and painful jaw could foreshadow an oncoming heart attack. Saliva flow and consistency is used to determine conditions such as dysbiosis, hormone issues and stress. After various examinations are completed, I interpret the findings and a program is designed according to the specific needs of each client.

Interpreting What Is Seen in the Mouth

According to a 2010 study from the Medical University of South Carolina in Charleston, up to 20 percent of patients with inflammatory bowel disorder develop lesions in their mouth that may even precede abdominal symptoms such as cramps and diarrhea. When I observe swollen lips and ulcers on the inside of cheeks and lips—a white centre with a red halo circling—I suspect Crohn disease once gum disease is ruled out. Often after many assessments, patients visit their physicians, who order lab tests that always confirm my suspicions.

If the lining of someone's mouth is very pale—a light shade of pink—I usually suspect anemia, a condition in which the body doesn't have enough red blood cells circulating. The tongue can also lose its typical bumpy texture and become smooth looking.

In acid reflux, stomach content regurgitates into the esophagus and mouth can dissolve tooth enamel and create erosive lesions near the back of the mouth that can be detected easily. Some individuals with acid reflux conditions recognize an uncomfortable heartburn symptom, but some patients may experience it only while they sleep and may not know they have it.

It's common for patients to say they're having trouble sleeping and not knowing why they're waking up in the middle of the night. Signs of stress patterns and gumline recession is also detected by examining the mouth. Most individuals are aware of when they are going through a very stressful period, but their mouth may indicate stress is taking a more serious toll than they realize. Many people grind their teeth, this is a condition known as bruxism and is a response to stress, which can wear down and chip your pearly whites. Many clients will say they are not teeth grinders, but most patients tend to do it at night while they're sleeping. We can detect all the telltale signs of mouth stress.

Periodontal Disease and Osteoporosis

Bone disease has no symptoms, which means most people don't know they have it until they suffer a bone fracture or take a bone-density test. An annual trip to the dental office may be just what your bones need before it's too late. Osteoporosis does not cause changes in the teeth, but it does cause changes in the bone supporting the teeth, which is part of the periodontal structure. This may show up as a receding gum line and loose teeth. And bone loss in the mouth typically means there are signs of bone loss elsewhere in the body.

Heart Disease and Periodontal Disease

Swollen, red and bleeding gums may be a telltale sign of heart disease. In fact, gum disease may put you at risk for both coronary artery disease and heart disease because the bacteria could travel to your heart and form blood clots or build up plaque in your arteries, which can impede your heart's blood flow. People with periodontitis and even early gum disease may often have risk factors that not only put their mouth at risk, but their heart and blood vessels, too. Risks associated with periodontal disease span A to Z, including Alzheimer's disease. They are too many to be included in this chapter. But in the case of Alzheimer's, evidence shows if you have oral and gut inflammation, your brain will also be affected. See more in the bibliography.

Oral Cancer: The Sobering Facts

It is not my intention to digress or to distress the reader, but I would like to point to the fact, oral cancer has overtaken cervical cancer as the most common HPV-related malignancy in the United States. It is the sixth-most-common cancer in the United States. Regular dental visits can help catch signs of it in its earliest stages when survival rates are more than 80 percent. According to Canadian Cancer Society statistics in 2017, 4,700 Canadians were diagnosed with oral cavity cancer and in the same period 1,250 Canadians died from oral cavity cancer.

When actor Michael Douglas candidly revealed his throat cancer was linked to having oral sex, two things happened. He made headlines that mortified his family. And he helped publicize the fact that a pervasive, sexually transmitted virus called HPV was unleashing an epidemic of oral cancer.

An oral-cancer examination is a part of dental examination and is always done as part of a dental-wellness evaluation in my practice. My clients are aware they are making an appointment for a wellness evaluation, not "teeth cleaning and a check-up." For more information, visit my clinic website at www.integrativehealth.info or www.drsheilamckenzie.com.

Orthodox Treatment of Periodontal Disease

The standard orthodox periodontal therapy will usually consist of the following.

Scaling. The removal of soft and hardened deposits from your teeth above and below the gum margins and gum pockets and root planning, which is smoothing the root surfaces to enable the gum tissues to reattach to your teeth.

Curettage. The soft-tissue lining of a periodontal pocket is scraped away to help the gum tissues heal by forming new tissue.

Gingivectomy. This is a surgical procedure in which deep pockets are eliminated, leaving a shallow crevice that is easier to be maintained by the patient. This is done when the disease does not involve the jaw bone.

Flap Surgery. Gum tissues are opened surgically to gain access to deep pockets and roots to remove calculus. The gum is then sutured back into place. Sometimes the bone around the tooth is reshaped, or part of it is removed.

Antibiotics. Antibiotic therapy for periodontal disease is quite unnecessary, in my opinion. Dr. Farghen, a dentist in Sarnia, Ontario, echoes this statement in an Ontario dental journal. I quote: "Antibiotics are often inappropriately prescribed." Often missing in this one-leg approach is attention to systemic support. It is as if the mouth is detached from the rest of the body.

Holistic Approach

In addition to removing the infection in the immediate area of the mouth, a sensible holistic approach optimizes nutritional therapy, immune support and detoxification protocols are integrated into the program for the best outcome of the client's health. My approach is to design a program geared to the specific need of each client

.

This chapter is offered to provide basic information as to how the reader can start a Self-Care-in-Action© plan. I would like the reader to understand that detoxification, health maintenance and restoration is not complicated. Many of the healthcare providers would like you to believe health is complicated, with thousands of diseases requiring thousands of drugs and trained experts just to keep you alive.

I would like to reassure you, health is very simple because the body was designed to function for a lifetime. All living things, including microorganisms, owe their lives to the creator's blueprint, not medical intervention. The suggestions I offer here will decrease inflammation, support your immune system and enable your microorganisms to work in a symbiotic relationship. These are first-line, effective, basic techniques I have used and experience excellent result with my clients for many years. I also provide more specific add-ons and homeopathic immune system support, according to each client's needs.

The basic part of this program can be easily adapted by the reader and will pay big dividends in your overall health:

Keep Your Mouth Clean

Correct techniques for brushing and flossing can be found on my clinic website which is provided in the resource section of this chapter. Do not use any commercial toothpaste and mouthwash that have a high alcohol content. Gargle can be used to rinse debris from your mouth and throat and help to soothe pain and decrease inflammation. Another important function of gargle most often overlooks is it allows nutrients in the gargle to be absorbed in the mucus membrane of the mouth before reaching the stomach and intestine. This is another reason why alcohol mouthwash should never be used.

Echinacea and Enzyme Gargle

Grind one to two uncoated chewable papain tablets, into a powder, then mix with 10 drops of echinacea and add to an eight-ounce glass of distilled water. Take a mouth full and gargle for about thirty seconds, then swallow and repeat until the glass is empty.

Enzymatic and Vitamin C Gargle

Grind one to two chewable papain tablets into a powder, combine the powder with one-half teaspoon of calcium ascorbate, or magnesium ascorbate crystals or powder, add to four ounces of distilled water, stir until completely dissolve, gargle with a mouth full of the mixture for thirty seconds, repeat until the container is empty.

Torrens Tooth Powder

Combine 1-part sea salt or Epsom salt with 6 parts baking soda. Place in an electric blender and close lid. DO NOT add water. Put on high speed for 5 minutes. Leave lid on for another 5 minutes while powder settles. Place in a sealable jar. Dry brush your teeth, then wet finger and dip in mixture and pat powder on gums and let sit for 5 - 10 minutes. Rinse with warm water. Repeat daily.

I often recommend topical application of Vitamin C. As stated earlier, gum-disease symptoms are like vitamin-C-deficiency scurvy. In fact, it is like having small wounds all around your teeth. Vitamin C boosts wound healing in general and integrity of periodontal ligaments and works as an anti-inflammatory.

Remember, you should not use pure ascorbic acid on your teeth. You must use a non-acid form of vitamin C known as "calcium ascorbate." It is safe to leave on your gums. You can pour about a teaspoonful in the palm of your hand and use a wet finger to pat it onto the gum margins. You can keep it on for ten minutes and spit it out without rinsing, but if you dislike the metallic taste you can rinse with a small amount of warm water.

Fine Tune Your Diet

Reduce simple sugars (white sugar, honey, fruit juice and refined carbohydrates (flour and pastries) from the diet as much as possible. Emphasize flavonoid-rich foods such as berries (blueberries, blackberries and hawthorn berries). Eat as close to a vegetarian diet as possible, cultivate good bowel habits with fibre to cultivate probiotics and reseed the gut from time to time with probiotics. Limit your consumption of meat and stop eating foods with, chemical-laden food additives.

Monitor Your Saliva

Normally, saliva has antibacterial properties that keep your mouth clean and your breath fresh. When you aren't drinking enough water, your body becomes chronically dehydrated and stops producing saliva. Your mouth might not be totally dry, but you're not making enough saliva to kill the bacteria. Some people experience bacterial overgrowth and as a result, their breath stinks.

White and Clumpy Saliva: Candida fungus can cause a yeast infection in your mouth, which is also known as "thrush." Candida begins in the intestinal tract and eventually moves into the stomach, up to the esophagus and finally into the mouth. Depending on how thick the yeast becomes, it can be seen in the mouth and on the tongue. The fungal yeast mixes with the saliva, turning it white and clumpy.

All you need to test for excess yeast or thrush is a glass of water. For six days, when you wake up (before you eat or drink anything) spit a dime-sized amount of saliva into a six-ounce glass of water. Watch for changes in your saliva in the water over a 45-minute period and write down your results each of the six days.

If your saliva stays floating on top, candida overgrowth is likely not an issue for you. If it grows legs, then candida is likely an issue and could be getting in the way of your hormonal and whole-body health. This is a sign it's time for a tune-up. If it sinks to the bottom of the glass, you'll want to get this under control as soon as possible, check bowel frequency increase fibre and water and take probiotic supplements.

There are two ways to increase the accuracy of this test: Do not consume dairy the day before you start testing or on any of the six days, as it can thicken the mucosal membranes and give you a false positive. Stay hydrated, as dehydration can cause your saliva to sink and result in a false positive. If you suspect you have yeast overgrowth, follow the dietary suggestions and use probiotics to re-establish gut flora.

Dry and Sticky Saliva: Dry and sticky saliva could indicate you suffer from sleep apnea. This is a common disorder whereby you experience one or more pauses in breathing during sleep. Breathing pauses can last from a few seconds to a few minutes. They may occur thirty times or more an hour, according to the National Heart, Lung and Blood Institute (NIH). Usually, normal breathing resumes with a loud snort or choking sound. Sleep apnea is chronic. As a result, the quality of your sleep suffers.

Unfortunately, sleep apnea is often undiagnosed since doctors can't detect the condition during routine office visits. A Chinese study conducted on sleep apnea patients found those who were at high risk for developing cardiovascular disease produced less spit than those who were not at high risk.

Here Are My Basic Supplements for an Anti-inflammatory and Health-Building Technique

In addition to taking a general multiple vitamin and mineral supplement appropriate for your gender, I also suggest taking systemic enzyme, Systemic enzyme therapy is used to decrease pain and inflammation in the gum and support the immune system. I suggest papain (enzyme from papaya fruit), take 250 mg 3x daily on an empty stomach for systemic action and a general digestive enzyme with 3 meals. You need to saturate the system with five key nutrients; water, niacin, vitamin C, carotene and sulfur.

Niacin Saturation

Niacin saturation is indicated by a mildly warm ear and facial vasodilation of blood vessels often called "the flush." Take niacin, also known as vitamin B3 (not niacinamide), every ten to fifteen minutes until you feel the flush. Start by taking 50 mg and increase to 100 mg, then continue taking enough niacin throughout the day so each dose makes you feel a slight bit warmer. A flush should end in about ten minutes, if it lasts thirty minutes and you feel a bit spacey, you took too much, but it is totally harmless. A large dose of niacin on an empty stomach will result in too long a flushing action, so take your niacin right after a meal.

Since niacin is a vitamin and not a drug, it does not require a prescription and it is not addictive. Niacin is sold in any pharmacy or health-food store. A good rule when taking niacin is to take all the other B vitamins as a complex, separately, in addition to the niacin. Vitamin B12 is poorly absorbed in the digestive system the best method of B12 except for injection is intranasal (by way of the nose). Buy ready to use over the counter Vitamin B12. Capsules. Open the capsule and apply the contents inside the nostril with a clean finger or Q-tip. Be gentle and please remember not to put a whole capsule in the nose. The idea is to coat the inside of the nose.

Vitamin C Saturation

How do you saturate with Vitamin C? Take it until you are symptom-free. The effective level is known as the "saturation level" or "bowel-tolerance level." Gradually increase your daily dose until you have or are on the verge of having diarrhea. Remember Vitamin C diarrhea is not dysbiosis

Dame Dr. Sheila McKenzie, RDH, PhD, DHMS, DHS

diarrhea, which is frequent, watery and explosive. Cut back slightly and remain at that saturation level.

Carotene Saturation

Juice a basket of dark green vegetables and orange colour vegetables, such as carrots, twice daily. When your skin turns orange, you are at saturation level. This is called "hypercarotenosis" and is completely harmless. Juicing also ensures you are fully hydrated; vegetable juice is preferably over plain water. In addition, juicing provides you with a lot of trace minerals. Beta carotene from vegetables is converted to Vitamin which is essential for healthy, mucus membrane, immune system and vision.

Sulfur Saturation

Research shows low sulfur diets appear to contribute significantly to the drastic increase in illness or to the slow and ineffective rates of recovery, premature aging, dependence on all types of medication, autoimmune diseases, skin disorders at all ages, poor skin tone and colour, autism, viral and bacterial infections, circulation and heart problems, allergies, arthritic pain, increased incidents of flus and health annoyances, some mood disorders. The drastic deterioration of our overall sense of well-being appears to be influenced by and related to the low sulfur. I consistently used organic sulfur at the saturation level as part of my inflammatory protocol for many years with remarkable results.

It is best to follow an acclimatization period, especially if you have any food sensitivities, allergies, or environmental illness. It is very important you begin with a low amount and gradually increase to the recommended amount. In a few situations, the gradual increase can take up to two months, although it is usually three to four weeks.

For a healthy person weighing 120 - 150 pounds (54 - 68 kilograms): Take half a teaspoon of organic sulfur once a day in the early morning for four days, then increase to half a teaspoon twice a day (early morning and about nine hours later) for four days, then increase to one teaspoon twice a day (same times) for four days. If there are no flu-like symptoms to indicate a healing crisis, go with the recommended amount for your weight and health issues. While coping with stressful situations you may increase your daily amount. See Resources, below, on where to get organic sulfur.

Homeopathic Minerals

As I stated earlier homeopathic prescription is most effective if done by trained homeopaths after taking into consideration your constitution and genetic predisposition, but in general homeopathic tissue mineral is readily available and is inexpensive and I highly recommend them for self care. Calc Fluor 12X (Calcium fluoride) may strengthen tooth enamel, both Kali Phos 6X (potassium phosphate) and Kali Mur 6x (potassium chloride) have been key Tissue Salts to support healthy gum.

Here are some general reports I received from clients who adhered to this protocol: no more bad breath or bleeding gums; teeth appear whiter; firm, healthy gum tissues; no more pain in the face or jaws; no more headache or neck pain; no more depression; weight loss; being able to cancel surgical procedures; clearer thinking and improved mental energy; and overall feelings of well-being.

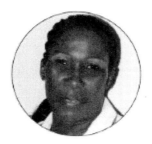

About
Dame Dr. Sheila McKenzie, RDH, PhD, DHMS, DHS

Dame Dr. Sheila McKenzie, RDH, PhD, DHMS, DHS graduated from the Jamaica Ministry of Health, Dental training program and worked with the ministry of health school dental health program before immigrating to Canada. In Canada, she satisfied qualifying examination for registration with the Royal College of Dental Surgeons of Ontario (RCDSO), as a registered dental hygienist (RDH) in 1981.

Early in her practice, she decided an integrative medical approach to healthcare delivery was best for her practice and to this end she continued studies into various health disciplines. Her broad base postgraduate training enables her to integrate many healthcare specialties in a unique oral and systemic healthcare practice. She has accumulated numerous credentials which include, doctor of homeopathy, an integrative medicine doctor, internal medicine diploma and many diplomas and accolades.

Dame Dr. Sheila McKenzie has delivered numerous international and national lectures and conferences, appearances on Tv and radio and written articles in magazines. She was appointed and served as a minister of health and health ambassador under the International Parliament for Safety and Peace for ten years.

Recipient of numerous awards including, Harry Jerome award for Health and Science, Markham Mayor's, outstanding citizen in the Markham community, the founder of Clinics for Humanity™, current president of the World Organization of Natural Medicine, knighted under the Sovereign Order of Orthodox Knights Hospitallers, for her humanitarian endeavours. Dame Commander for Ontario region and Health ambassador for the Orthodox Order of Saint Paul, head of the Department of Natural and Humanitarian Medicine at Saint Peter and Saint Paul Lutheran Institute -

Lutheran University and Chancellor of the Canadian College of Humanitarian Medicine.

Resources

For more information, visit my website: www.drsheilamckenzie.com or www.integrativehealth.info.

My book: Eclectic Home Medicine Cabinet By. Dr. Sheila McKenzie, is available on my website www.drsheilamckenzie.com.

I have good results in using organic sulfur from: The West Coast Organic Sulfur http://www.organicsvulfur-msm.ca.

References

1. Smith LH, Clinical Guide to the use of Vitamin C (Summary report of Dr. Frederick Keller research paper) Caranza E Glickmans's Clinical Periodontology, W.B. Saunders, Philadelphia, 198 Tacoma, WA: Life Science press, 1972

2. Vimy MJ Lorscheider, Fl. Intra-oral mercury released from dental amalgam, j. Den Res 1985; 64, 1069 - 1071.

3. inorganic mercury World Health, Geneva, 1991. Perspective of Amalgam and Other Dental Material, (Friberg L., Schrauzen G. Nieds) Stultart, Thieme, Verlag, 1995 in press.

4. Christen A., The Clinical Effects of Tobacco on Oral Tissue, JA BA 198,81 pp 1, 3, 78 - 82.

5. Bastaan R. and Reade R., The Effects of Tobacco on Oral Tissue, Dent J.1976, 21pp, 308 - 15.

6. Pelletier, O. Smoking and Vitamin C Levels in Humans, Am. J. Cin. Nutr. 1968, 21pp, 1259 - 67.

7. Association between dental health and acute myocardial infarction, Malbla, K.J. et al British Medical Journal, Vol. 298, March 1989, pp 779 - 782.

8. Periodontal Disease and Cardio Vascular Disease, Beck, J.D. Presented at the symposium of the "Relation of Periodontal Infection to Systemic Disease". Journal of Periodontology, Vol. 67, October 1996, pp. 1123 — 1137.

9. Alvanes, O., Altman, L. Springmeyer, S. et al. The Effective Subchemical Disease in Nonhuman Primates, J. Periodontal, Res., 1984, 16pp, 628 _ 36.

10. Krause, M. and mahan, L. Food: Nutrition and Diet Therapy, W.B. Saunder, Philadelphia, PA, 1984.

11. Brenton G. and Ingold, K., Beta Carotene, an Unusual Type of Lipid Antioxidant, Science 1984, 224 pp 569 - 73.

12. Freeland, J., Cousins, J. and Schwartz, R., Relationship of Mineral Statusand Intake to Periodontal Disease, Am. J. Cin Nutr, 1976, 29pp 745 — 9.

13. (eds), Trace Elements in Dental Disease, John Wright PSG Inc., Boston, MA, 1983, chapter 9 pp 99 — 220.

14. Hazan, S. and Cowan, E., Diet, Nutrition and Periodontal Disease, American Society of Periodontal Dentistry, Chicago, IL 1975.

Chapter 6

Miraculous Healing Through Pure Spiritual Intelligence

By: Mr. James MacNeil

Are You Ready for Your Miracles?

Congratulations on your commitment to your optimal holistic health. I trust you are devouring the genius insights from all the chapters in this incredible compilation of wisdom from gurus. I'm honoured to be included.

Holistic health includes the holistic-health mindset of mind, body and spirit and yet goes deeper to include soul and heart (not just the one that pumps blood). It acknowledges the synergistic reality of the whole rather than simply the wellness of each individual dimension.

We Don't Actually Know What This Physical Body Can Do!

You've likely heard of, or can easily research, health miracles from around the world. I'm referring to the immediate and irreversible physical healings from all sorts of illness and disease, as well as the mystical "flying yogis" and those who have mastered surviving on sunlight instead of food. Sceptics may rightly disprove some of these "wonders" as advanced parlour tricks, but more importantly, some defy our current scientific explanations. I want you to enjoy truly miraculous health!

Who Am I?

I believe you will be well served by having a clear visual map of your true and complete personhood.

You are a creative and compassionate spiritual being currently living in a physical form in this time/space continuum. You are perfect in your personhood, exquisitely unique and infinitely valuable and your natural state is in euphoric connection to "SourceLove" and all living things.

"You Don't Have a Soul,
You Are a Soul. You Have a Body."
Made famous by C.S. Lewis

Your soul is who you are! You have a spirit, a mind, a body and a heart (non-physical). Please note that four of the five dimensions of "you" belong to the spiritual world and only your body exists in its natural environment.

The main differences between the spirit world and this time/space continuum, for our purposes here, are as follows:

- The spirit world transcends time, so it's always NOW.

- The spirit world also transcends space and matter, so mapping our soul, spirit, heart and mind is a little tricky.

- The spirit world has no negativity, like fear or frustration, so there's a beautiful flow of faith.

What Are the Roles and Responsibilities of Your "Parts"?

Your soul is "who you really are," and the most important thing is to remember that!!!

Your spirit is your connector to SourceLove and all living things.

Your mind is your "thinker" and "knower." It is in charge of making sense of and managing, the gap between the spirit world and this physical time/space continuum. It uses your brain when you are thinking consciously.

Your heart is a unique level of consciousness. It is your centre for all action and attraction. It perpetually plays the dual roles of servant and master. In the wisdom literature we read, "Guard your heart above all else, for it determines the course of your life."

Your body is... your body.

The following illustration is a map of "The Real You." Take some time to meditate on this image and its truths.

For more information on The Real You, please accept, as my gift, a downloadable copy of my book Pure Spiritual Intelligence and a full coloured version of the image above at tinyurl.com/PureSI.

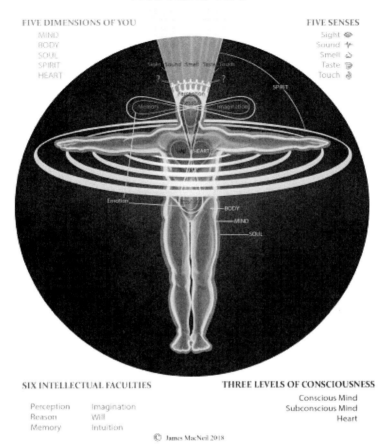

THE REAL YOU

FIVE DIMENSIONS OF YOU

MIND
BODY
SOUL
SPIRIT
HEART

FIVE SENSES

Sight
Sound
Smell
Taste
Touch

SIX INTELLECTUAL FACULTIES

Perception	Imagination
Reason	Will
Memory	Intuition

THREE LEVELS OF CONSCIOUSNESS

Conscious Mind
Subconscious Mind
Heart

© James MacNeil 2018

Energy, Thought and God

Before I complete my brief description of The Real You, specifically the importance and power of your six intellectual faculties, I want you to become familiar with the workings of energy, thought and God in this time/space continuum.

This universe is made up of one thing: ENERGY. Energy can neither be created nor destroyed. It not only permeates all things, it is the substance of which their parts are formed. Energy exists in perpetual motion and is always moving from highest concentration to greatest dispersion, except when employed for creation. I'm referring to the second law of thermal dynamics, entropy: all things move toward disorder. Therefore, at all times, you are creating or disintegrating.

Creation, for us, begins with THOUGHT. Thoughts are things, actual things. Thoughts are our first creation, because they are the drawing together of energy. This new thought is an energy ball and it immediately becomes a new cause in this universe of cause and effect.

The power of this new "thought thing" is expanded through the addition of emotion and compounded through repetition. The most obvious effect of this new thought is the feelings it provokes within our bodies. Because of this new thought, we immediately begin to vibrate at a new frequency, which affects our mood, mindset, wellness, actions and attractions. There is an ever-growing body of evidence that proves definitively thoughts, feelings and words powerfully and measurably affect our cells and our environment.

Since my chapter is on miraculous healing, let's agree to agree on the topic of GOD, SourceLove, Source Energy, Ki, Chi, Allah, Infinite Intelligence, the Universe and for my Star Wars fans, the Force. We may not agree on the name, or the religious methodology of connecting with this entity or energy, but almost 100 percent of us can agree there's something, if not someone, beyond our capacity to comprehend.

My research has led me to believe we all have a sense there is something, and we all seem to have, on some level, a desire to understand and/or connect with this something or someone. Every religion is simply the best set of ideas, actions and/or the clearest path to this peaceful connection that an individual or group of individuals has organized.

I personally believe this something is a someone who is 100 percent cool with you, without any rituals, mantras, or animal sacrifices. That's my belief. I respect and learn from all religions because I find golden wisdom in all of them. In an attempt for full disclosure, with no overt or covert intent to persuade or offend you, I am a fully committed Christ follower with a strong aversion to religion. My discomfort with religion is based on my belief that its existence perpetuates the false belief that there is a gap between us and God, which I believe does not exist. Do you still love me?

If we are, in fact, primarily spiritual beings living temporarily in this time/space continuum, we can and should align with our spiritual power for miraculous wellness. I've created the term "SourceLove" to represent this spiritual force, from which this entire time/space continuum was created, in an attempt to serve all who, read this, including you, so they benefit from these truths without undue distractions.

SourceLove transcends this time/space continuum yet exists within it and permeates it, as energy. We connect with SourceLove through peaceful presence, thereby tapping into the limitless supply of clean-burning fuel, as the sun feeds the plants and we co-create with SourceLove through thought.

Intellectual Faculties, Infinity Loops and Manifestation
The birthplace and "build place" of thought is our intellectual faculties. They are memory, reason, imagination, perception, will and intuition. These faculties are interlocked in infinity loops, which build on their creative power, fuelled by emotions and perceptions and thereby compound their impact.

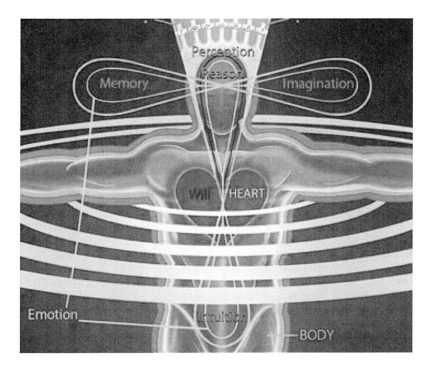

The most important insight for holistic health is the relationship between the intellectual faculties and the heart. The heart is the centre for all action and attraction, which is the trigger for perpetual manifestation in your physical body and in the world around you.

> *"As a Man Thinketh in His Heart, So Is He."*
> *Proverbs 23:7*

How Do I Acquire Miraculous Holistic Health?

Miraculous holistic health is your natural and normal state. You need not create, conjure, or force optimal health onto yourself, but merely return to your natural, happy, healthy, wealthy and wise equilibrium. Please embrace these facts:

You are a creative and compassionate spiritual being, currently living in physical form in this time/space continuum. You are perfect in your personhood, exquisitely unique and infinitely valuable and your natural state is in euphoric connection to SourceLove and all living things.

> *You are perfect in your personhood, your design is perfect and*
> *if you there is any negative truth about yourself, it is either not*
> *true or not negative.*

The first and most important fact about our wellness, wealth, happiness and legacy is we are plug-ins. Our natural state is riotous connection to SourceLove, from which our miracles flow. We are spiritual beings and cutting ourselves off from the spirit world robs us of holistic health. If a kettle, intended to boil water, was never plugged into its power source it could still be very useful, but its true purpose and power would never be revealed or experienced. When we are peacefully connected to our source, we immediately and eternally experience the three super vitamins of love, joy and peace, which heal and empower us.

Your peaceful path to power starts with being fully present and at peace with your current reality. The most common methods for reconnection are:

- Uninterrupted time in nature
- Meditation and/or Prayer
- Time with newborn babies or animals
- Agenda-free time with loved ones.

76

The ancient wisdom literature uses a special word for the state of disconnection from source: "Hamartia," which translated into today's English, means sin. I understand the word is not popular today, but in ancient Greek, the uses of the word included "missing the mark" in archery and the "tragic flaw" in a theatrical character. These uses have given birth to the modern misconceptions of the word. From its root words, Hamartia simply means not-together, or separation — like a tree robbed of sunlight would experience a waning of wellness.

It's truly that simple to tap into the universal-miracle energy. Jesus said, "I have come that you may have life and life more abundantly." He was referring to "Zoe life," which refers to a limitless, uncontainable, miraculous, flow-of-life energy, like a mighty river into which we simply fall and enjoy the ride of miraculous wellness.

How Do I Protect and Perpetuate Miraculous Holistic Health?

Regarding environment, nutrients and rest, my peers are the leading experts on this and I happily defer to them for these insights. The only element I would stress in this dimension is the idea of the sabbath. The sabbath is the spiritual discipline of rest. To prioritize the time required for rest requires faith that you can afford the time. Strategic rest, intended to reconnect with SourceLove through reconnecting with nature, meditation and prayer, allows our mind, body, soul, spirit and heart to return to the natural perfect rhythm and flow.

Regarding the mind/body relationship.

1. Thoughts are things

Energy balls, that can grow and have profound effects on the cells of your body and therefore your wellness. With this in mind, you can now understand why virtually all the thought leaders, preachers, teachers and knowledge-for-profit professionals echo, at the top of their lungs, "Mind your mind!" Make a commitment and a conscious, deliberate, determined effort to nurture positive, loving, gracious thoughts and imaginings.

'Fix your thoughts on what is true and honourable and right and pure and lovely and admirable. Think about things that are excellent and worthy of praise."
Philippians 4:8

2. Beliefs give birth to all miracles and manifestations

Beliefs activate your heart's action-and-attraction mechanism and unlock your miracles and manifestations. A belief is an unchallenged feeling of certainty relating to a thought. Your thoughts are things, energy balls, that grow in size and strength with emotion and repetition.

When they hit the critical mass of unchallenged confidence, they form a belief. It's of urgent importance that you realize as long as a belief is held in your heart and mind, it is your self-created destiny. This is a fact, whether your beliefs are love-based and life-giving or based in fear or frustration, which robs you of Zoe life, love, joy and peace and severs you from SourceLove and all living things. Beliefs are like blocks in the brain—building blocks or stumbling blocks—so choose wisely!

3. Metabolize life experiences!

When your physical body takes in food, whether healthy, appropriate food or the least-healthy junk food, it always seeks to metabolize these new resources. It will *use,* s*tore* or *eliminate.*

- **Use** - Make the most of the moments in life by practicing pure presence. Pure presence is a form of Nen consciousness, or One Mind. (In contrast to Zen consciousness or "No Mind".) Nen is the egoless practice of being fully engaged in the moment and fully detached from its outcome. This is also, in sporting terms, referred to as "the zone".

- **Store** - Meditate on your life experiences to draw out the insights and wisdom.

- **Eliminate** - Sadness and grace are our toxicity-release mechanisms. Allow the natural and appropriate grieving process to release the negative aftermath of challenging life experiences. This is one of the most important disciplines of a holistic healthy life. Within this elimination process, you are freed from negativity through intentional and appropriate sadness, forgiveness and repentance.

I hope, pray and trust you will enjoy pure, holistic health in riotous connection to SourceLove and all living things. Please know and remember, you are a creative and compassionate spiritual being living in physical form in this time/space continuum. You are perfect in your personhood, exquisitely unique and infinitely valuable. Be the blessed blessing you are

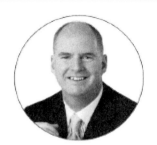

About
Mr. James MacNeil

Mr. James MacNeil is a Best-Selling Author and the Founder of Verbal Aikido, Guru Builder and Dream life GPS. He is one of the world's most accomplished speakers having addressed more than 2,000 live audiences and having shared the stage with mega brands including Les Brown, Tony Robbins, Larry King, Bob Proctor, Steve Forbes, Rudy Giuliani, Robert Allen, T. Harv Eker and Sir Richard Branson.

For more information on The Real You, please accept, as my gift, a downloadable copy of my book Pure Spiritual Intelligence at: tinyurl.com/PureSI.

Chapter 7

Holistic Diabetes Wellness

By: Cheryl Ivaniski,
D.Ac., C.H., RDH

10 Life Changing Principles for Preventing, Repairing and Healing Diabetes

Diabetes is so common it has become a household word. It is a condition that affects the human body on every level. It touches every tissue, organ and cell in the body and knows no boundaries. It can be very subtle and silent as in my Grandma's case. She struggled with diabetes experiencing the ill effects of high and low blood sugar levels for more than 42 years, until it eventually took her life. Those with diabetes are affected with a shortened lifespan by 5 - 15 years on average compared to those who do not have diabetes.

It diminished her vision until it stole her eyesight, it caused neuropathy, tingling, pain and numbness in her limbs, it affected her legs, ease of movement, mobility and her ability to walk. It robbed her of her energy and enthusiasm for doing things she would have loved to do more of in her life, as well as her independence. It eventually affected her mind, now classified as Type 3 Diabetes. We now know there are several more types of Diabetes. Grandma had Type 2 and 3 Diabetes.

Diabetes can also come on quickly. For a few weeks, I had not been feeling well. I was not just overly tired, I was exhausted and my body was constantly agitated. Little did I realize my body was shutting down and my organs were dying. I recall vividly as though it was yesterday exactly what had happened to me when not one, but two life-giving organs and glands blew out. I was keynote speaking to hundreds of doctors, dentists and health care professionals at the Toronto Convention Centre when the ceiling was spinning so fast, like the most thrilling ride at your favourite theme park and the floor was swirling from out underneath my feet. I was so dizzy and I could feel the room going velvet black, completely dark. That is the last thing I remember. I was immediately rushed to the hospital in a semi-comatose state. It was totally unexpected. It abruptly hit me and came out of nowhere. The Doctors told me days later how lucky I was to be alive and the testing showed my blood sugar numbers were above the highest recordable numbers.

My pancreas had shut down completely - it had gone bankrupt. In fact, I learned this was not something that was going away and not something I could recover from. This was a huge shocker ... and it didn't stop there, that is not all. It got worse. At the same time, my thyroid gland completely shut down, so now it was not just one organ that had failed me, but my gland at the same time. My thyroid gland blew out having only a trace of thyroxin.

Neither was functioning and I was told they would never function again. I often ask myself if I had worn them out being a type 'A' personality that was on the go, go, go and just never stopped. Now I would have to really look at my life and assess how I was doing things. At this point, I had no choice. Having Type 1 Diabetes where my pancreas produces no insulin, requires me taking as many as 5 - 9 injections per day or a continuous way to deliver insulin into my body - through an insulin pump which acts as an artificial pancreas. Without insulin, those who have Type 1 Diabetes do not usually live beyond 7 days on average. This is a very serious condition that requires attention 24/7 every day.

This led me on my new journey. Because I lived in a family with active Type 2 Diabetes for as long as I could remember, this meant I also witnessed the many complications of diabetes. My family was very obedient and followed all the directives from our Dr.'s. Even though all suggestions were followed, this still did not halt the complications of diabetes from affecting my grandmother.

Maybe you, a family member or loved one is having this same experience. Even though I asked the doctors and nurses questions about a more preventive approach and for anything they thought that could help me to improve my health and help avoid these devastating effects, they always gave me the same common answers, the best resource is to take the hospital program. I did, in fact, I did it multiple times and I just shook my head thinking, that's it? You have got to be kidding,

Although I am very grateful for traditional medicine for keeping me alive, it was not contributing to preventing potential complications. Witnessing what my grandmother went through every day in her life, I was not about to follow or accept the devastating and predictable future of complications. I was looking for a more preventive and proactive approach and that was not something that was offered or even available.

Remember, I come from a very physically active, hard-working family who were farmers in the country who grew organic vegetables, chickens and fruit. I had a solid upbringing of being healthy. I was also trained traditionally in nutrition, pathophysiology, histology and understood cellular health and cellular damage. It was in that very moment, I knew there just had to be more.

Without knowing how, I made the decision to make it my life's mission to take on how to support my body, nourish my mind and start winning with Diabetes. That is when I made the choice to take 1,000 % responsibility to learn all I could. This led me back to university where I earned my Doctorate in Holistic Medicine and Acupuncture. I learned how the body heals and all about energy medicine. I started applying these modalities in my life and there was a noticeable improvement in my blood sugar levels and overall health. This led me to study and apply so many other therapies.

My preventive options were growing by leaps and bounds. I indulged in applying them in my life and in my private practice with patients. This is when people suffering everyday started feeling relief and hope. They felt understood because not only am I a licensed professional, I am someone who truly relates to how they feel because I have those exact same challenges . . . so I get it ... totally. This really fueled my soul and inspired me in helping more people.

The chronic effects of high blood sugars are the reason for so many of the complications affecting hundreds of millions of people worldwide. If you have diabetes or know someone with diabetes, you know exactly what I am talking about. It robs you of your energy and stamina. It affects the joy in your life and your enthusiasm. It affects your mindset and decreases your interest in doing things and participating fully in activities. It affects ease of movement and mobility, your finances, future retirement savings, your independence and most of all, your quality of life and longevity by 5 - 15 years.

High blood sugar levels are super stressful on the body and this plays havoc contributing to the imbalance of your hormones. This in turn influences your mindset, often welcoming mood swings and depression. This in turn is often the time when Dr's prescribe additional medications instead of healing therapies to help you manage stress more effectively. I feel this is the time for you to learn new tips and tools and principles to nourish your mind and body.

371 - 425 Million people worldwide are affected by diabetes. Diabetes is no longer an epidemic. It is a global pandemic. 187 million people do not even know they have it according to the International Diabetes Federation. The thing is, about half of you have yet to be diagnosed and are walking around in life not even knowing you have pre-diabetes or that you are borderline. If you have a tendency towards diabetes, you are best to start

being proactive right now because this is your best chance of living your best quality of life.

For those of you who have pre-diabetes, especially, you have the most power to do something about it before it develops into diabetes. If you have prediabetes, you are at a higher risk for acquiring diabetes, or if you have or had gestational diabetes, you can prevent getting Diabetes.

If you have Type 1, 2, 3 or 4 Diabetes, I am here to help you enhance your quality of life and longevity. It is because I have learned and continually learn new exercises and practices that I apply in my life and I know you can apply in your life too. Now, I get to share them with you. I create custom programs that are body friendly and promote healing.

If you would like to find out more about how you can start living your empowered life and start feeling the benefits of nourishing your body mind and soul, contact me. I walk with you every step of the way so together we create your own customized program for you and/or your family members and your clients if you are a health practitioner. Many practitioners who want to make a positive difference in the lives of their clients can also contact me. Sometimes practitioners add this specialty to their growing practice. Visit
www.lifestylewellnesscentre.com or www.diabeteswellnesscentre.com.

Diabetes is relentless and knows no boundaries affecting your body, mind and spirit. It is overwhelming and can easily and subtly over power you. I am here to say, it is time for you to take a stand for your healing and take your power back. It is time for you to be victorious, to truly live your best life and to start thriving.

I believe healing is taking all the best information and best practices that we know and combining the best of traditional and natural medicines together offering the Holistic (Integrative) Approach to healing your body on all levels. I do not believe healing is any one practice or about discounting any one discipline.

But What is Diabetes?

I believe it is very important to understand how diabetes works in the body. Most people suffering with this disease are not given the vital information they need to make better choices for themselves. There are medical definitions of diabetes, which leave us powerless, so let's have a conversation that is much simpler and more relatable. This way we have a new way of understanding diabetes and gaining power with what else is possible.

My definition: is one that allows you to understand not only what it is, but how it affects you. When your body lacks insulin, or the cells used to produce, receive and transport insulin malfunction (meaning they do not work at all or they work at an impaired partial capacity) the sugar broken down from the foods you eat has no choice, but to spill into your blood stream. It has nowhere else to go. Because sugar is not supposed to be in your bloodstream, it is toxic to your body and it contaminates, disables and attacks your nerves, tissues, organs and cells eating away at them causing inflammation, breakdown and death. This is why there are so many devastating complications of diabetes. Each time our blood sugar numbers are even slightly elevated damage is occurring.

Facts and statistics show us that diabetes is the leading cause of blindness, kidney failure, non-traumatic amputations and it leads to at least 70 - 80% of heart attacks and strokes. We know it robs you of your energy and it welcomes mood changes, influences hormonal issues, depression and weight gain. These are all very real and devastating side effects of diabetes.

Now, I am here to tell you there is good news. I believe you now have a choice, if you want one. There have been studies including the DCCT (Diabetes Complications and Control Trial), in fact, it was stopped early because the effects were so amazingly positive when good blood sugar control was practiced. With all the healing practices there are today, I want to share with you that it is up to you to take a stand for your own health. You have the choice to be the active participant in your own healing. I am here to share with you 10 proven principles you can start integrating in your life right now that will make up to an 80 - 90% difference in your quality of life moving forward.

Take a moment, close your eyes and imagine what your body, mind and soul feel like with consistently normal blood sugar levels? How does your body feel? What is your energy like? What is your enthusiasm like? What would you be doing differently? What do you look like?

You have the power to give your body what it needs when it needs it, so it can function with normal blood sugar levels. Would you like to feel fully energized? Most people are living in so much fear and without any real healing plan. Without one, you are single handedly inviting all the complications of diabetes in your life both knowingly and unknowingly. I am here to take the guess work out of the, "What should I do question?"

I am here to share the 10 Principles to Living Your Life Vibrantly Well. My purpose is to give you the tools and strategies you need, one at a time, so you can apply them in your life and enrich our quality of life starting today. The immune system needs to be strong no matter what health challenges you have. This is the only way your body can defend and heal you. The body is remarkable and I want you to experience remarkable healing. Would you like to learn how to put a harness on the progression of your inevitable health challenges? Whatever health challenge you have, diabetes or something else, nourishing the body and mind produces positive results and helps you heal.

I want you to start winning with your health. You have the power to heal, you just don't know it yet. You have needed this piece - this life-giving information that you have been missing and this is your chance to join my community. I want you to join others and learn. I give you the strategies and tools that show you how you can be powerful in the face of diabetes. All you need to do is decide if you want to choose to start being victorious in your healing or become a statistic of the complications. Do you choose a healthier path for yourself or a continually exhausting and stressful path? The choice is yours.

I AM HERE TO SAY THERE IS HOPE. I AM HERE TO INSPIRE YOU IN YOUR JOURNEY IN HEALING YOUR BODY, MIND AND SPIRIT.

The Top 10 Principles for Living an Enhanced Quality of Life
1. Mindset - Mindshift

It starts with your mindset and being open to how else things can be for you. That may look like slight mind shifts over time or it may look like a bigger mind shift to start with and continual shifts over time . . . it is a process and is ongoing.

Knowing the devastating complications and severe effects diabetes has and the effects of other immune system challenges, the only question you need to ask yourself is do you want to go along in your life and be a victim like the hundreds of millions of those who have complications, or do you want to make a positive shift in your life, enhancing the quality of your health, healing, happiness? Do you want to have your independence, energy and more of your hard-earned money for you now and in retirement?

Mindset. Do you believe you can create what you want in your life? Do you believe there are other approaches you have not tried or are not aware of that may in fact influence positive healing for you? Sometimes it is the approach you need and then the steps on how to apply them. Why do some people heal so much better than others? What are they doing differently? This is where I come in.

As I watched my grandmother and so many others lose their sense of self and their everyday abilities, it affected me greatly as a young girl, teen and mature woman. I see what many of you go through in your life and that truly is unacceptable to me. I personally do not want to experience anything less than what is possible for me. I believe there is so much that is preventable and so much that can be reversed and healed.

My mission is to inspire, empower and educate you in such a way that you live with the heightened awareness on all levels (mind, body, spirit) knowing you get to live an enhanced quality of life that supports healing and longevity if you want to. Check out my chapter in Success Starts Today with Jack Canfield (available on Amazon) that shares with you how to have a healthy mindset. http://cherylivaniski.successstartstodaybook.com/

2. Emotional Release Work and Healing Trapped Emotions

Unreleased negative emotions cause stress on the body, adding to the stress experienced by diabetes. It wears your body down, overworks your organs every time you have even a slightly high blood sugar level and releases chemicals that cause complications. This is not what you want. The healing in your body needs to include your emotions as well.

There are many causes of emotional stress, including abuse, hurtful relationships, career and financial stress. In fact, entire books have been written on the subject. Unfortunately, it is not something that can be addressed in a few short words. Emotional healing is a journey for each person and each person works through issues differently.

If you feel you want more information or a new modality, I highly recommend you check out people like Louise Hays of Hay House Spiritual Healing and Dr. Bradley Nelson, creator of the emotional code and body code. Both are experts in their field and will help you to overcome the damage caused by unresolved emotions.

3. Nature and the Outdoors

Nothing is better than mother nature. There are many places and then there are special places on this earth that help bring healing to the body. One of my favourite places is in Sedona, Arizona. There are electromagnetic fields that encourage balance and healing and it is a very powerful place to spend time to enable healing. Magnet therapy, crystal and gem therapy, tapping, walking and hiking in the woods, being around trees, mountains and water, in gardens, around animals are some examples of healing environments. These are very good examples of being in nature.

4. Something Beyond Yourself - Spiritual Wellbeing

Listen to your body, attune to your body and become your own intuitive in your healing process. Learning how to become present in your body is like exercising a muscle, it takes practice and patience. You can learn how to become present in your body with such things as dowsing, applied kinesiology, meditation, visualization, yoga, practicing mindfulness, Tai Chi, Qi Gong and many other techniques teach you how to distress and develop your own intuition. I also offer spiritual coaching, as well as workshops and retreats. Visit www.lifestylewellnesscentre.com and www.diabeteswellnesscentre.com

5. Food - How We Fuel Our Physical Bodies

What you eat, your food choices, how you eat, portion size, the number of times you eat per day, how you combine your foods, the quality of your foods, etc., these all determine if you are making your body struggle and work harder, thus stealing your energy, or if you are helping your body to lighten its work load, giving your heart, digestive organs and other body systems the break and support they need to help healing occur.

Here are some things to consider:

- Quality of food - where it comes from (organic or processed)
- Food choices
- How we combine what we eat
- How much food we eat and what our body can process at one time is critical

90

- More items throughout day verses one or 2 big meals that the body cannot break down effectively = harm to the body where sugar is forced into the bloodstream
- Foods to avoid that shut down and make our body struggle stealing our energy
- Foods that encourage healing
- Glycemic indexes and their role (the rate - how fast a food raises your blood sugar)
- No more than 3 teaspoons of sugar at a time and why?
- Quality and amount of fibre
- Micronutrients and macro nutrients
- Vitamins and minerals (deficiencies and excesses.)
- Gut health and colon health, using digestive enzymes, prebiotics and probiotics
- How we prepare food, examples: boil, steam, poach, broil, fry, air fry, raw, etc.

Check out www.diabeteswellnesscentre.com for great checklists and recipes that will help you on your health journey.

6. Alkalize Your Body while You Hydrate, Hydrate and Hydrate

Your health largely depends on the pH level in your body. The ideal pH level of blood being around 7.4 is slightly alkaline and healthy. Did you know disease can only live in an acidic environment? Disease cannot live in an alkaline environment. Does it stand to reason you would drink water and eat foods that alkalize your body and avoid ones that toxify your body?

The reason this is so important for you if you have any health issue, pre-diabetes or diabetes is as soon as you have inflammation anywhere in your body and/or your blood sugar levels are higher than the normal range, then your body is fighting with itself and this produces acid. When this occurs, that acidity travels through your bloodstream throughout your body, causing those unnecessary silent, subtle damages that over time cause complications that are life debilitating and deadly. It is very easy for you to start taking an active role in your health. You take action.

7. Movement - Helps your entire body and all conditions, especially those with Diabetes and Insulin Absorption - Big Time.

Keeping your body active, keeping your muscles and connective tissue in communication is very important. It is particularly important for those with diabetes because with insulin resistance and/or not producing enough insulin. Either way exercise can help reduce the glucose in your bloodstream, which is the leading cause of why you have or will have complications. When you exercise, your muscles get the glucose they need and in turn, your blood glucose levels go down. It really is one of the most efficient ways to help control your blood sugar levels. Exercise also helps with keeping your arteries clean, helping to prevent blocked arteries which lead to heart and stroke problems. It also helps you maintain good cholesterol levels.

Additional benefits of exercise are:

- Lower blood pressure.
- More effective weight management
- Increased level of good cholesterol
- Leaner stronger muscles
- Stronger bones
- More energy
- Better sleep
- Stress management

Some examples of great physical exercise choices include: walking, biking, hiking, swimming, jogging, tennis, volleyball, basketball, skiing, zumba and dance classes, yoga classes, pilates, strength training and resistance exercises.

For those who love sports and obtaining more cardio in your life, indulge yourself and enjoy it.

8. Social Interaction with Others

It is more likely for you to suffer from health problems associated with diseases such as diabetes when you live a more isolated lifestyle and experience loneliness and thus generally more life dissatisfaction. It is important to maintain your physical and mental health at all ages. Being engaged with others where you are interacting and socializing stimulates your mind and body. It helps with a more positive attitude. Being socially engaged reduces dementia and ill effects of disease. Socializing can be the most important element in one's longevity.

9. Stress Management

There are many types of stresses you deal with or fail to deal with effectively without even realizing it. Stress on the body affects all systems, including muscles, respiratory, cardiovascular, endocrine, gastrointestinal, gut health, etc. Stress on the body causes muscles to tense up which can cause pain. Stress often results in tension headaches, neck and shoulder pain, neuropathies, arthritis, back pain, fibromyalgia, poor healing, skin issues, sleep disorders and leads to other chronic pains.

Respiratory stress studies show that an acute stress, such as the death of a loved one can trigger asthma attacks in which the airway between the nose and the lungs become constricted this can lead to hyperventilation and bring on panic attacks, anxiety and overwhelm. This same stress can overload the body throwing it into overwhelm triggering Type 1 diabetes. The cause of Type 1 diabetes is unknown, although it is thought that a virus or a sheep's liver fluke from the cow's milk may be a stress on the body that causes the pancreas to attack itself. It is an autoimmune disease. Overstress to my body is what I believe trigger this for me. It has been stated that toxins and bacteria - yeast in the liver and gallbladder can be a cause of diabetes.

10. Open Flows of Energy in Your Body

Keeping the Chi (energy) flow moving is most important. Some practices that enrich the circulation and improve energy flow in the body include: walking and body movement and exercise in general, massage therapy, acupuncture, acupressure, Qi Gong, yoga, aromatherapy (essential oils), light therapy, shiatsu, infrared sauna therapy and homeopathy to name a few.

The Choice Is Yours

My goal is to introduce you to the holistic approach to diabetes wellness. There are many practices and combinations of wellness therapies that naturally help you normalize your blood sugar levels consistently. It is with these therapies and integrating daily healing lifestyle choices that you will be able to prevent, repair and yes, even reverse some of the complications of diabetes.

If you want to skyrocket your energy, enhance your circulation, affect change in your vision and empower your body to heal itself, I am here to help. I want you to learn the top things you need to avoid right now, starting today and what you need to do more of right now to help you to start your healing process.

Come To:
www.lifestylewellnesscentre.com and www.diabeteswellnesscentre.com where you will learn the Top 10 Strategies that work together in guiding you in Reclaiming Your Health. Online coaching programs are available that go deeper into these principles along with a Step by Step Guides to living your most vibrant life. Come and join my community. To get access to my 7 Day Kick-Start Program and Access to my Master Class on How to Start Healing Your Diabetes Today for Free. Just Mention this Book. See you there.

Let This be a Healing Day in Your Life,
Cheryl Ivaniski, D. Ac., C.H., RDH

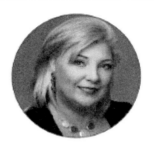

About
Cheryl Ivaniski D.Ac., C.H., RDH

Cheryl Ivaniski D.Ac., C.H., RDH is a Best-Selling Author, Speaker, Dr. Holistic Medicine and Founder: Lifestyle Wellness Centre and Diabetes Wellness Centre

Chery is the Best-Selling Author of her book "Success Starts Today" co-authored with Jack Canfield, New York Times Best Selling Author of Chicken Soup for the Soul Series. She's an award-winning author who has co-authored books with the World's Top Motivational Speaker Les Brown, Dr. John Gray, Brian Tracy, as well as Raymond Aaron.

Cheryl is a health authority, wellness advocate, Dr. Holistic Medicine and a professional, inspirational speaker who travels internationally sharing her expertise. She is a Wellness Coach who coaches organizations and people in living a vibrantly well life.

She hosts online programs and live events including seminars, workshops and conferences. She leads retreats, teaching people how to live the Enriched Diabetes Lifestyle. To invite Cheryl to speak at your event or for radio, tv and media interviews please contact her at: www.diabeteswellnescentre.com.

Chapter 8

Your Relationship Rescue Reset

By: Mr. Jim Hetherington

Eight Principles to Check Your Attitude About Relationships

Using the word ATTITUDE as an acronym, let's examine eight principles that, when applied to our lives, will bring a fresh new way to look at our relationships and marriages and ourselves. This will in turn, keep us leaning toward being the best version of ourselves we can be. It's not a one-time task, but rather an ongoing system that can be applied methodically to keep us on track.

When you get stuck in your relationships, as with everything else, you want to hit Reset and continue.

Let's have a look at the first letter.

A is for Adjust

Have you ever wondered what it would have been like to live in another time or era?

At some point most of us have probably wondered what life would have been like if we had been born in a different country or a different time. Perhaps even in a completely different culture. Or how about into a different socio-economic situation?

When we do this, however, we lose perspective on where we are and we don't really invest in the life we have or the relationships around us. We can start to blame the environment or our parents or our economic status for everything that isn't right. Then, we can slip into believing people around owe us something. We can rationalize — if I was born into the wrong place, then it's the world's fault and somehow it needs to give me whatever I want or need.

Far too often, we settle into thinking if only our circumstances were different, if only we had more, if only the other person (or the people around us in general) would treat us better and listen to us, things would be different.

The reality is the only place we can start to make things better is right here. Where we are right now is the only place to start. There is no option to be reborn in another era, time or economic bracket. The stork didn't make a mistake. We are here for a reason and a purpose. And the only people we truly have the power to change and control is ourselves.

99

What we need to do is adjust our attitude toward the people around us and take responsibility. We need to realize we are not the greatest gift to the world of relationships or marriages. If we spent half the energy working on ourselves, as we do complaining or working to change others around us, things would be a lot different. We would become people whom others want to be around.

What if we got into the habit of getting up each day, looking into the mirror and saying, "I'm going to be the best person I can be today"? Don't let the world dictate what your day is going to be like — you decide. Decide to make your day and yourself, better in the process.

If you struggle with having meaningful relationships, take a new approach. Instead of pursuing other people, do everything you can to be the person people want to pursue. Look for ways to adjust.

T is for Think

From the time we were born, we began the process of thinking.

I'm sure our first thoughts were, "What am I doing out here! I was warm and cozy and now strangers are touching and handling me in this strange new world."

Parents or guardians started by communicating with us, challenging us from an early age. They spoke to us and challenged our thinking; they played games with us and read books to us, all to make us think. As we got older, we started to develop the ability to reason and began thinking on our own. Many of the references we keep in our minds come from these early stages when people were challenging us to think.

Time to time, as we grew up, situations arose that hurt us or caused us offence. Our brain remembers those events and forms systems to help protect us. For example, most of us have had an encounter with a hot stove or boiling water. We may have touched one or the other and were stunned by the feeling. Our brain remembers that and from then on, we know not to touch anything hot.

When we get into a disagreement with a partner or friend, what is the first thing that comes to our minds? Usually it's a recollection of a similar event from our past. We say to ourselves, "This is just like the last time" or "This is what happened before and this is how I responded." The old thinking kicks in to guard and protect us. What we need to do is look at the situation and evaluate things from a new view and ask ourselves, "Do I need to respond as I did before? Should I deal with this the old way? What new approach should I take? Is there something in me that needs to change?"

One of the dangers I see with getting older is we can forget to think and apply new thoughts to a situation. We simply allow old patterns to take over and we follow their 'advice' without challenging them.

My suggestion is to look at each situation and rather than respond by default, look at the response you're about to make and ask if this is valuable to you now—should you respond differently? Examine the response, recognize how it came into being and see if a new way can be introduced as you move forward.

Challenge your thinking!

T is for Talk

Talking is an incredible tool. Unfortunately, in relationships, men and women have two different approaches. For women, it's automatic to share and to express feelings and ideas. They can verbalize things more easily than men. Psychologists tell us women have about 20,000 words a day that they need to share and men have a need to share about 5,000 words a day. There are exceptions, of course, but generally speaking, it comes more naturally for women to share and talk.

Men may not know how to share. Culturally, boys are raised to be rugged, not to cry or share emotions. Men are seen as weak if they cry or want to talk about their feelings. So, when they enter into a relationship, if they don't change their mindset, they will go on to be quiet and non-expressive. Women want to share their feelings and know what is going on most of the time.

Remember when men process things, they get quiet and think. Women like to talk right away, men usually don't. When they're ready to talk, they will. It's important to respect each others' process. In relationships we need to take a new approach to talking. We must understand that keeping things inside doesn't help us physically or emotionally. We have to acknowledge just thinking about things will not bring true understanding to relationship issues or concerns.

Go to my website, www.yourrelationshiprescuecoach.com, for a powerful exercise that couples and friends can use to learn to communicate more effectively.

With practice you can be a better communicator. So many relationships and marriages fail because of the inability to communicate. If we stop trying to be right in every situation and listen to the other person, communication would become more effective.

If you're going to fight, why not fight for each other? Fight for the person rather than against the person. Have your friends' and partner's back.

I is for Invest

The principle behind an investment is whatever you put time, energy or money into will, over time, grow. For example, if you take five thousand dollars and give it to a bank to put into a GIC (guaranteed investment certificate), after a period of time, when the certificate matures, its worth will have increased.

This principle can be applied to relationships!

Just as there are many ways to invest money and different levels of risk, there are several different ways to invest in relationships. They will cost something and may be risky. However, there are huge rewards to be had for those who invest wisely and risk a little.

Some people don't want to risk getting hurt, or losing, so they don't invest. They'd rather stay at home and play video games or watch TV than take on the risk in relationships. I would suggest we take a good hard look at ourselves and know who we are before we start searching.

Now let's talk more about long-term relationships—not classroom friendships or work relationships, even though these can grow. If we want to attract the person we desire, we need to know two things.

First, who we are. We need to know what we value, what we stand for and what the real deal breakers are for us when it comes to a partner. If we don't have a strong understanding of who we are, then anyone who comes along will do. If they don't fit our future plans and goals and if they don't value the things we do, then it's irrelevant how good they smell or nice they look.

Second, who they are and what they stand for. What are their goals and plans and where do they want to be in ten years? If you meet the most attractive person ever, but they don't line up with your values or plans for the future, why would you want to invest in a long-term relationship? What kind of investment would it be? The return will be little to none. Get to know them. Who they are, what they believe and where they are going.

And remember there is risk. There is a chance of being hurt or rejected. However, if you take the time to know who you are and what you really want and then begin to search out like-minded people, if you go slow and let things develop and evaluate things as you go, the risk will be less. It's when people rush in without thinking and without a plan that things can and usually do, go very wrong very quickly.

As with any good investment, be wise and do some research. Do your homework up front and the payoff will be huge. Without doing the homework, you may just have to settle for less or stay in and continue to play video games.

This T is for Trust

This is a huge area. Almost every person has an area where they lack trust in something or someone. But because we are relational creatures, most of us do want to trust.

When we were young, a friend may have stolen something from us or a bully may have taken something that belonged to us. Maybe, when we were young and innocent, somebody took advantage of our heart and broke it. Or perhaps someone in our close circle of friends abused our trust or did something to damage our reputation. The result could be that, as we grow up, we lack confidence in people. We find it hard to trust. This can be carried into adulthood.

As you get to know a person and see their values, directions and goals, you lower your guard a bit and allow them to enter into your circle of trust. Little by little, as you get to know each other, the guards come down, until you are in each other's trust circle. If you let your guard down too fast, you risk being too vulnerable. If you let your guard down and they don't, it's the same thing: you become vulnerable to being overexposed. If the surrender isn't mutual and doesn't happen at the same time, the balance can be thrown off; trust isn't reciprocated.

Going back to the idea of having your own values list, knowing who you really are will certainly help in the trust area. If you aren't confident in who you are, it may be impossible for you to trust anyone or for anyone to trust you; know who you are and what you stand for. Don't go back and forth on ideas and values; know who you are and where you stand. As you exude confidence, you can receive it from others and walk in trust.

In my training seminars I spend more time dealing with and reconciling past wounds. As we deal with them, we can move forward to see things in a new way. We gain a greater expectation for the future. For more information, go to my website,
www.yourrealtionshiprescuecoach.com.

Go slow when you're getting to know others. Let them prove to you that you can trust them; don't just throw your heart wide open and hope for the best.

U is for Undo

Take a look at the areas in which you have problems with trust and begin to reflect on how you can undo those areas. Start with undoing limiting beliefs.

Limiting beliefs will keep people trapped like nothing else. The self talk that goes on in our head can defeat us before we even have a chance, a real chance, to succeed.

Too many people have little confidence in themselves. Many don't have the ability to operate at an optimal level. And the sad thing is many don't even know it! They have no idea, because these beliefs are the norm for them. Because it's all they know, that's all they do.

If you think negative, you will become negative. If you think you're bad at something, you will be. If you think you're not very good or not very smart, you may never become great or experience the benefits of being intelligent.

Henry Ford said whether you think you can or can't do something, you're right. If you think you will never be able to do a particular task well, or you'll never get good grades, you're right. The decision you make about something will become your reality. Stop thinking in the negative. Undo that thinking and start moving forward in the positive and make a change. Make a difference. Having healthy and happy relationships is a skill. Being able to relate with people well is a skill, something we need to work on everyday.

How do we make these shifts? By replacing the old habits, the old mindsets, with new ones. By replacing the negative talk with positive talk. By speaking powerful and positive affirmations over and over. And by being consistent. Make it a daily habit to grow and learn. Write down your negative talk and write out what you will say instead. Post affirmations in your bathroom, your office—anywhere you will see them—then repeat them over and over.

I take my coaching clients through a five-step process to overcome limiting beliefs. If you want to learn more, sign up for a free session and discover how this process can help you at:
www.yourrelationshiprescuecoach.com.

Undo limiting beliefs and make that shift.

D is for Determine

We need to look at our relationships. We need to decide how important they are to us. Then we need to decide how we will make our relationships grow and how we will invest in them.

It takes time and energy to form good relationships and good marriages. The more energy we put into a relationship, the more successful it will be. If we put little or no time into it, we will get no value from it. So, we need to determine how important relationships are to us.

We can all have good relationships, but we need to determine how much energy we're going to put into them and what relationships we want to invest in and why.

Motives for building relationships can be very different. We might want to have a relationship for companionship or friendship. These relationships are strictly relational so we have someone with us. In these relationships we share special interests. It could be sports, it could be a hobby, it could be a club, or it could be our school or work experience and so on. These relationships are strictly for companionship—to have a friend and to have someone to socialize with.

We can also have romantic relationships. These relationships are more serious, a place where we have a deeper connection. These relationships are very important, but we need to be aware of them as we go.

There may be several reasons for us to have relationships and we need to determine what they are. We need to determine what values we place on each relationship. In order for us to be a good friend, we need to know ourselves first. We need to examine our hearts and know if we are motivated by selfishness. We need to examine our hearts and determine how much energy we're willing to put into a relationship and if it's for the person or something we will gain from them.

We need to keep ourselves in a circle of friends who will challenge us. Les Brown, the motivational speaker, once said, "If you're the smartest person in your circle of friends, then you need a new circle of friends." Friendships and relationships provide comfort and encouragement and support. But they are also meant to challenge us. They should challenge us to be the very best person we can be. If they aren't challenging us, but instead, are taking us in an unhealthy direction, we need to get out of that circle.

In my book *Your Relationship Rescue Handbook*, I have eleven "F" words I use as a framework for individuals to figure out who they are and what they believe in. It's also for couples to use so they can share the same core values in their relationship. To find out more, go to www.increasethelove.com.

E is for Example

Examples need to go both ways in our lives. We need to be an example to those around us and we need to have people set examples for us.

To be successful in relationships we need to have people in our life who can be examples for us to follow, people we can look up to and say, "I want to be like that." They're role models. They're mentors. They're the people who take us to the next level. Without people in our lives to emulate, we will stay the same. Without a shining example, we would carry on and not be challenged to grow.

We may have younger brothers or sisters, or younger friends, in our lives. We may even have children. All of them will look to us to be an example of what a friend is to be and what a person is to be like in a relationship. Many of us learned what relationships are by watching people around us. Our parents were probably our earliest examples of relationship. We gained a lot of knowledge, without even being aware of it, just by watching others as we grew up. They could have shown us a good or bad example — either way, they set examples that we learned from as we matured.

When we have people in our life who are good examples for us and when we are good examples for others, we become the best person we can be. When we operate at our highest level, we draw others to their highest level, too.

If we don't live as an example for others, we might keep them from moving forward and reaching their fullest potential.

The eight principles we looked at here can be applied daily and used as tools to help you become the best person you can be. Remember to write down what you believe, what you stand for and begin to attract that kind of person to you. And remember to take responsibility for yourself and become the best possible version of yourself and encourage others to rise up to be their best.

In my book, Your Relationship Rescue Handbook #2 - 8 Ways to Help Your Attitude, you can explore these principles further. If you found this chapter helpful you may want to check it out at www.increasethelove.com.

You can become a better friend and partner. By adjusting your attitude and hitting the Reset button, you will continue to be a person whom others will want to be around.

I wish you much happiness and success in all your relationships.

To Continued Health and Happiness!
Jim Hetherington

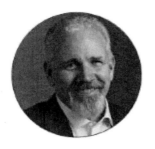

About
Mr. Jim Hetherington

Mr. Jim Hetherington is a coach, speaker and an award-winning author. He's passionate about working with individuals and couples to help them discover ways to have more meaningful relationships and marriages. Through his material he encourages people to see the value of having strong relationships in every area of life; personal, business and spiritual.

Along with writing and coaching, he also holds training events where he works with groups and leads them through valuable principles to challenge people to grow and to be more aware of who they are and how they interact with others.

Also, as a licensed wedding officiant in Ontario, he loves having the opportunity to work with couples to create a ceremony that reflects the couple's uniqueness. He has travelled to Central America over 15 times where he does short-term mission work. While there he teaches and does humanitarian work.

He has been married to his wife Mary for 36 years and they have two children together. He and his wife call each other best friends and enjoy working, travelling and spending time together.

If I can be of any further help, please reach out to me at: jim@yourrelationshiprescuecoach.com or visit my website to find out about other training and helpful articles

Chapter 9

Cancer Prevention and Treatment

By: Dr. Akbar Khan

A thirty-one-year-old female contacted our clinic for assistance. She had been recently diagnosed with the deadliest form of brain cancer, glioblastoma. This type of cancer carries an average prognosis of survival for a little over one year, even with all the best therapies, conventional medicine has to offer (surgery plus chemo plus radiation). Clearly, she understood the odds were not in her favour and decided to look beyond what was offered by her cancer specialists.

After finding our clinic and receiving a comprehensive consultation, we determined she was an excellent candidate for dichloroacetate, a drug that triggers natural cancer-cell death by depriving the cells of their main energy source, glucose. Unfortunately, this drug is not considered mainstream and is not approved as a cancer therapy, despite solid scientific evidence supporting its use in treating cancer.

The patient received a standard course of combined low-dose chemo and radiation from her oncology team. She declined further standard therapy, consisting of monthly high-dose chemo, due to real concern about life-threatening side effects. Instead, she started taking dichloroacetate, which is non-toxic. She received no support from her oncology team for this unapproved therapy.

After three months, the patient felt well. All therapy was stopped and she was followed closely by her doctors. She required no further cancer therapy and has had no recurrence of the glioblastoma over nine years later.

With difficult problems like cancer, we sometimes need innovative, out-of-the-box thinking. In this case, it involved the use of a science-based new and different treatment method. Although it may seem obvious that oncologists would quickly embrace safe and effective therapies such as dichloroacetate, in fact it is the opposite. In this chapter you will learn the truth about this reality.

Cancer Has Become the Most Feared Disease

Cancer is generally regarded as the most feared of all diseases today. A quick look at the World Health Organization's cancer statistics reveals this fear is not unfounded. The WHO states cancer is the second-leading cause of death globally and was responsible for over eight million deaths in 2015. This represents about as many deaths *per year* as the entire population of New York City.

Throughout the world, nearly one in six deaths results from cancer. Tobacco use accounts for nearly one-quarter of all cancer deaths. The economic impact of cancer is massive and increasing year after year. It is estimated the total annual economic cost of cancer in 2010 was about US $1.16 trillion.

Current Cancer Control Strategies Are a Failure

Given the staggering statistics on incidence (new cases of cancer) and mortality (deaths due to cancer), it is abundantly clear the current overall anti-cancer strategies are an abysmal failure. We have all heard the expression "prevention is the best medicine," yet with cancer the medical system continues to focus on treatment. Little effort is directed to effective prevention strategies.

What About Prevention?

Prevention can be broken down into two subcategories:

1. Primary prevention (stopping the disease from developing) and
2. Secondary prevention (early disease detection at a point when it is curable).

In our medical system, most of the cancer-prevention strategies are secondary prevention, which is also called screening or early detection. Primary prevention strategies are more effective than screening/early detection, yet primary prevention is poorly implemented.

This is easy to see once we break down the individual prevention strategies. Table 1 shows the currently available primary and secondary prevention strategies recognized by the Canadian Cancer Society.

Table 2 shows cancers that have no secondary prevention strategies. While primary prevention strategies apply to all cancers, clearly most cancers do not have well-accepted effective secondary prevention/early-detection methods.

Table 1 – General cancer prevention methods recognized by the Canadian Cancer Society (http://www.cancer.ca)

Primary	Secondary
Don't smoke	Breast screening (mammogram, examination)
Eat well	Colon screening (colonoscopy, fecal occult blood test)
Be active	Prostate screening (PSA, examination)
Maintain healthy body weight	Testicular screening (examination)
Limit alcohol	Cervical screening (Pap smear, examination)
Follow sun-safety guidelines	
Get vaccines (e.g., HPV, Hepatitis A, B)	

Table 2 - Cancers with no recognized secondary prevention (early-detection) strategies

Cancer Type	Secondary Prevention Strategy	Cancer Type	Secondary Prevention Strategy
Brain	None	Ovary	None
Bladder	None	Pancreas	None
Kidney	None	Sarcoma	None
Leukemia	None	Stomach	None
Lung	None *	Uterus	None
Lymphoma	None		

*High-resolution CT scans can be done, but this exposes the body to gamma radiation, which increases cancer risk.

Primary Prevention Applies to All Cancers

The primary prevention methods such as eating healthy and staying active do apply to all cancer types. Unfortunately, there is no comprehensive primary-prevention strategy across Canada and only passing emphasis on such strategies during a typical doctor's office visit. Doctors have minimal training in the use of therapeutic nutritional strategies and no time to discuss detailed diet plans with their patients. Doctors may wish to help patients attain a healthier body weight, but weight-loss programs are not funded by government health insurance.

Have you ever seen a doctor design an exercise program for a patient? This is a time-consuming endeavour. The current Canadian health system paradoxically rewards doctors who see many patients in a short period of time and provide minimal care. Fitness counselling is therefore rarely performed.

Are "Approved" Smoking - Cessation Strategies Really the Best?

Doctors have limited methods at their disposal to help patients quit smoking. Approved quit methods include nicotine-replacement therapies such as chewing gums and patches applied to the skin, which have high failure rates. Specific antidepressants are approved to reduce nicotine cravings, but they come with significant side effects such as sexual dysfunction and suicide.

One of the most effective anti-smoking strategies is the use of modern safety-tested electronic cigarettes that contain nicotine. Numerous published studies show their safety and effectiveness, yet Health Canada and the Canadian Cancer Society, oddly, take the position that electronic cigarettes are a danger to smokers and should be avoided. Meanwhile, e-cigarette lobby groups have formed to actively combat the false information that is being spread to dissuade smokers from trying e-cigarettes.

Sun Avoidance or Sunscreen Avoidance?

We know that moderating exposure to the sun can help prevent skin cancers. However, avoiding sun exposure and using sunscreen, in theory, has the opposite effect for all other cancers. Ultraviolet light from the sun reacts with the skin to activate vitamin D and numerous large studies show that optimal vitamin D levels in the body are associated with lower risks of cancer.

In addition, the first prospective cancer-prevention study of vitamin D has recently been published. This study goes beyond demonstrating an association between optimal vitamin D and lower cancer risk—it proves that optimizing vitamin D intake actually prevents cancer.

The Miracle of Vitamin D

Curiously, in Ontario, the government has stopped funding vitamin D blood testing. It's terribly disappointing to see Health Canada's guidelines for vitamin D dosing recommend a grossly inadequate 400 - 800 IU per day with no testing of blood levels. The guideline goes on to assert "there is no additional health benefit associated with vitamin D intakes above [these levels]." Nothing could be further from the truth!

This guideline is in direct contradiction with the available peer-reviewed research, which confirms vitamin D blood testing *is* required and optimal dosing is about *ten times higher*, at about 4,000 to 8,000 IU per day. The vitamin D studies show significant overall survival benefits from taking such "high" doses of vitamin D. Not a single pharmaceutic drug in existence can claim the improvement in overall survival that has been attributed to vitamin D when it comes to heart disease, autoimmune disorders, or cancer.

It is essential to keep in mind, vitamin D has a wide therapeutic window — in other words, a wide range of dosing that is safe and effective. No one should be afraid to take vitamin D doses in the range of 5,000 - 10,000 IU per day along with periodic monitoring of 25-hydroxy-vitamin D blood levels.

Are Mammograms Useless?

Regarding secondary prevention, the latest research on the use of mammograms indicates these tests are barely effective. A 2006 study of over 1,000 women found mammograms only contributed 7 percent to improvement in five-year survival compared to breast examination.

Also, there is a justifiable concern that repeated radiation exposure to the breast from annual mammograms may, ironically, contribute to the development of cancer. Furthermore, compression of the breast during the mammogram procedure can theoretically encourage the spread of cancer cells if a breast tumour is already present. False-positive mammograms can also lead to significant anxiety and unnecessary invasive biopsies.

PSA is Passé

Screening for male cancers may be equally ineffective. The PSA test is a blood test routinely used in Canada to screen for prostate cancer. PSA is used despite the fact that it has limited accuracy, yielding false positive results that frighten men into thinking they have cancer when in fact they may simply have an infection. Rectal examination is also used by physicians in an attempt to find early-stage prostate cancer. Such examination is limited, because the doctor is able to feel only those tumours that are at the posterior (back) of the prostate and close to the outer surface.

Why Is There Conflicting Information?

As a result of all the conflicting information available on primary and secondary cancer prevention, it is easy for the average person to become confused and make decisions that could profoundly affect their lifespan and quality of life. First one must understand why so-called medical experts and large, respected cancer organizations and charities deliberately spread half-truths and even outright lies.

The answer becomes evident if you follow the money. Prominent cancer charities receive significant ongoing donations from the pharmaceutical industry, so naturally they will do everything possible to support that industry. If they promote highly effective prevention strategies, this will lead to a decline in the use of very expensive anti-cancer drugs, which will result in financial loss for their donors. In other words, it pays to keep people sick.

Even Health Canada is not immune to conflict of interest. When they approve a new drug to be released to the Canadian market, a portion of the gross profits from the sale of the drug must be paid to Health Canada. This is not a fixed licensing fee, but a percentage of the profit. It is therefore no surprise to us that Health Canada firmly discourages Canadians from using the most powerful and effective cancer-prevention strategies such as high-dose vitamin D and nicotine-containing electronic cigarettes. Neither one of these requires licensing, so the revenue to Health Canada would be minimal as compared to that for a pharmaceutical such as a nicotine patch.

Appropriate Prevention Recommendations

Given the conflicting views on cancer prevention, driven by the goal of massive profits, it is imperative for individuals to avoid blindly following the direction of health "authorities." Instead, people should form their own opinions based on the current scientific literature.

Unfortunately, this is no easy task, since peer-reviewed medical literature can also be affected by various forms of bias. One can even find overtly false published studies, seemingly written with the goal to support the existing health industry, which depends on the public suffering from chronic diseases for their profits.

It takes an experienced scientist to dissect the medical literature and weed out the junk. That is exactly what we have done on behalf of the reader. Based on extensive literature review, combined with years of clinical experience, we believe the following are the most effective and simple anti-cancer strategies available today:

1. Take Vitamin D3 daily in appropriate doses (typically 5,000 IU or higher) adjusted according to the blood level of 25-hydroxy-vitamin D. **Note:** this applies to Canada; hot countries may be different.
2. Use premium-quality safety-tested electronic cigarettes with nicotine for smokers who are unwilling or unable to quit, combined with appropriate education on proper use of the device.
3. Implement a calorie-reduced diet that avoids large amounts of sugars, large amounts of red meat/processed meat/smoked meat and products altered from their natural state (e.g., by GMO, or hormonal manipulation) along with maintaining a healthy body weight.
4. Vaccinate individuals at risk of infections that are known to cause cancer (e.g., Hepatitis B vaccine for liver-cancer prevention and HPV vaccine for cervical, anal and oral cancer prevention).
5. Reduce harmful inflammation in the body (e.g., chronic infections and autoimmune disease).
6. Get regular aerobic exercise.
7. Maintain a healthy, diverse microbiome (bacteria living in the body).
8. Maintain a low-stress lifestyle.
9. Avoid environmental toxins and carcinogens in general.

Various factors listed above do interact and overlap. For example, maintaining an optimal vitamin D level will automatically help to reduce harmful inflammation in the body. Exercise may lower stress. Vaccination can prevent chronic infection/inflammation.

Even people who may be genetically predisposed to developing cancer (for example, individuals with many family members affected by cancer) can implement an *effective* cancer-prevention strategy. The reason is that gene expression (how genes are turned on or off) can be modified even if the genes themselves are fixed.

The process of modifying gene expression is called epigenetics. It may be surprising to learn that simple things can change how genes are turned on or off. For example, changes in diet, level of exercise and stress level can all affect gene expression.

This means we are not simply stuck with the genes we are born with. We have the ability to modify how those genes operate—thus we have the ability to effectively reduce cancer risk even if our genes favour the formation of cancer.

How to Implement a Prevention Strategy

Many of the listed anti-cancer strategies can be implemented without assistance. Vitamin D blood levels can even be tested at home with mail-in kits. Ideally, individuals should seek the assistance of a suitable medical practitioner to optimize their anti-cancer protocol. Oncologists do not focus on cancer prevention, so they are largely of no help in this situation.

Family physicians are ideally suited to implementing a cancer-prevention strategy, but they rarely have adequate time to spend on this and may be biased by incorrect guidelines that are designed to promote chronic diseases rather than prevent them. For example, most family doctors will advise following the current Canadian vitamin D guidelines, which can have the potential to do a great deal of harm to the patient.

The ideal practitioner is a naturopathic doctor, an integrative medical doctor, or an osteopathic doctor. In some cases, other medical practitioners, like chiropractors or extended-class nurses, may have received the appropriate postgraduate training to develop an effective cancer-prevention program.

A Quick-Start Guide

Even before seeing a suitable licensed practitioner, one can begin to implement a prevention program. Here is how to get started immediately:

1. Start taking a high-quality oral liquid vitamin D3 at a dose of 5,000 IU daily (within one to two months a vitamin D blood test must be performed and calcium blood level should be measured).
2. Smokers should start using a premium-quality electronic cigarette with nicotine and throw away their cigarettes. **Note:** For reliable education about electronic cigarettes, consult www.vape-md.ca.
3. Reduce the portion sizes of all meals.
4. Reduce the intake of all artificially sweetened items (soft drinks, coffee, desserts, etc.).
5. Ensure the consumption of red meat/processed meat/smoked meat is not excessive.
6. Start taking a high-quality probiotic daily (spore-based bacteria are excellent).
7. Start fifteen minutes of daily exercise (matched to your current fitness level).
8. Take a fifteen-minute break every day to do something relaxing and enjoyable (listen to music, meditate, sit in the garden, etc.).
9. Purchase a water-purification system (for example, reverse-osmosis) and use it to supply all household water used for drinking, cooking and making ice cubes.

All of the steps listed are easy to implement and highly cost-effective. Reverse-osmosis water-purification systems have come down in price recently and typically cost less than $300. Electronic cigarettes are much cheaper than tobacco cigarettes, vitamin D is very affordable and exercise is free!

What if I Have Already Been Diagnosed with Cancer?

If you have been diagnosed with cancer in the past or you are currently dealing with a cancer diagnosis, it's not too late to implement a prevention strategy. The reason is having a history of a prior cancer means increased risk of developing a new cancer in future. Also, many of the prevention strategies that have been discussed actually assist with cancer treatment as well.

Modern cancer therapy is based on three primary modalities:

1. Surgery (removal of tumours), which can be curative and also has many potential side effects depending on the type of operation.
2. Radiation therapy (high-powered gamma rays or proton beams), which can be curative in a very small number of cancers, assists with symptom control and has significant side effects depending on the region being treated—e.g., skin burn, permanent dry mouth, impaired healing, brain swelling.
3. Cytotoxic chemotherapy (drugs that kill all rapidly growing cells in the body), which can be curative in a small minority of cancers, contributes little to long-term survival in adult cancers and has many severe side effects, including disability and death.

Other modern treatment categories include:

1. Hormonal therapy (blocking natural hormones that can encourage the cancer to grow; for example, breast and prostate cancer), which is not curative and has side effects, including immediate menopause, bone loss, muscle loss, poor concentration and fall in libido.
2. Targeted therapy (drugs that target a specific protein on the cancer cell to stop its growth, reduce its spread, kill the cell or prevent the formation of blood vessels in a tumour), which has multiple serious side effects that vary depending on the drug.
3. Immunotherapy (activating the immune system to kill cancer cells), which has serious side effects, including organ destruction by immune over-boost and increased rate of cancer growth.
4. Ablative therapy (using heat, cold, or electric currents to destroy tumours — e.g., RFA, NanoKnife), which is relatively safe.

Despite exponential advancements in medical science, cancer continues to be a major killer. WHO statistics show the number of cancer deaths is increasing. It is disappointing to see that, even though billions of dollars are spent each year on research, we are not having much of an impact on cancer deaths.

The high number of deaths can be explained in part by the increase in new cases of cancer diagnosed every year. So the next question to ask is: are we making an impact on cancer survival? In other words, are the current allopathic medical treatments allowing cancer patients to live longer? And if so, by how much? The WHO provides some thought-provoking data that shows the mortality (death rate) from adult cancers increasing steadily from

1950 to about 1990 and then gradually falling in recent years. However, the death rates are now roughly the same as they were in the 1950s and '60s.

It is interesting to note that the rates of smoking in several countries with the largest populations have been falling since the 1980s (India, China, USA). Could it be the reduction in smoking rates that has caused the improvements in cancer mortality and *not* modern advances in cancer therapy? No one knows for sure, but it is certainly plausible.

The Real Benefits of Toxic Cancer Therapy

Most people have a friend or family member who has been diagnosed with cancer and has undergone some form of allopathic cancer therapy. The public is aware of the horrors of chemotherapy: vomiting, hair loss, weakness and general decline in health.

Chemotherapy drugs are also the most powerful immune-suppressing drugs used in the practice of medicine. Since we know the body's immune system plays a vital role in the elimination of rogue cells like cancer cells, it certainly seems counterintuitive to treat cancer with immunosuppressive agents.

A group of doctors in Australia decided to examine a large body of chemotherapy research to see if chemotherapy really saves lives or if we are just reducing tumours only to have patients die from chemo's side effects.

The study question was: what is the contribution of chemotherapy to long-term survival in adult cancers? The researchers looked at randomized clinical trials of chemotherapy that reported five-year-survival data in the USA and Australia. The result of this 2004 study was shocking. The overall contribution of cytotoxic chemotherapy to five-year-survival in adults was *less than 3 percent.*

Based on the dismal survival benefits of chemotherapy, the authors concluded "a rigorous evaluation of the cost-effectiveness and impact on quality of life is urgently required."

One may assume the oncology community would take notice and make major changes in the use of chemotherapy in treating adults with cancer. However, nothing has changed in fourteen years. Chemotherapy remains the major modality of treating adults with cancer that has spread (or is likely to have spread microscopically). Clearly, our so-called evidence-based medicine is not so evidence-based when it comes to the use of chemotherapy. The profits from administration of chemotherapy are too great to suddenly drop this therapy.

Critics may argue this was only one study and the findings may therefore not be accurate. However, when we look at individual clinical trials of chemotherapy for various cancers, we find the data to be similar (a minor survival benefit from the therapy, such as a few weeks or months). Or worse, we find an absence of survival data. This means adult patients who suffer through harsh chemotherapy, hoping to be cured may in fact be receiving minimal or no actual survival benefit.

For this reason, it is the authors' opinion that we must look at novel systemic (whole-body) cancer therapies that address the root cause of cancer formation and growth, namely disordered cell metabolism.

Data continues to be published that supports the idea that cancer is not a genetic disease, but a metabolic disease. It is now felt that cancer cells are formed when the energy-producing units of healthy cells (the mitochondria) are damaged by environmental factors (toxins, infections, etc.). The mitochondrial damage leads to genetic mutations and uncontrolled cell growth. Various experiments have proven this theory, but most of the oncology community continues to believe cancer is primarily a genetic disease (caused by broken genes). Perhaps this misguided belief (leading to the lack of acceptance of metabolic cancer therapies) is the reason oncologists are getting such poor results, since they continue to focus on treatment strategies developed in the 1950s.

It has now been established by published human-case reports that metabolic cancer therapy is effective and also safe (e.g., publications on dichloroacetate use in humans). It is unfortunate that metabolic therapies like DCA don't attract research funding. We believe the main reason is the drug is generic (off patent) and cannot be sold for large profits. The effectiveness and safety of the therapy seems irrelevant.

In addition to DCA, there are many other generic drugs and natural medicines that have been shown to effectively treat cancer in humans. None of these drugs will be adequately researched and approved as cancer therapies as long as our current profit-based research model dominates the cancer industry.

It is time to look beyond billion-dollar profits and accept new, effective methods of cancer treatment based on generic or natural medicines that are available for human use today. The fastest way for this to happen is for cancer patients to take action. Patients must learn the true risks and benefits of the therapies offered. If there is no data to prove that a highly toxic therapy improves the odds of survival, or the survival benefit is minimal and patients systematically refuse to accept such therapies, the industry will have no choice, but to change.

The patients hold the power. Now they must exercise their power for the benefit of the current and future generations.

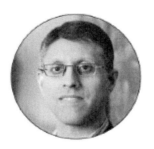

About
Dr. Akbar Khan

Dr. Akbar Khan is a graduate of the University of Toronto, Faculty of Medicine (1992). He completed his certification in Family Medicine in 1994. At the start of his career, Dr. Khan worked as an addiction consultant and research supervisor at the Addiction Research Foundation in Toronto (now called the Centre for Addiction and Mental Health). Dr. Khan has also been actively involved in pain and symptom management for cancer patients since completion of his medical training.

Through this work he developed an interested in cancer treatment and improvement of quality of life. In 2006, Dr. Khan, co-founded Medicor Cancer Centres, the first integrated private cancer clinic of its kind in Canada. Since 2007, Dr. Khan has gained international recognition for his work with off-label drugs in cancer treatment. Dr. Khan was the first in the world to demonstrate the curative potential of dichloroacetate when used as an adjuvant to radiotherapy or chemotherapy and the first in the world to publish on the benefits of intravenous dichloroacetate for cancer treatment.

In the last 3 years, innovative cancer prevention strategies have been added at Medicor, with a focus on vitamin D, natural medicines, nutrition and smoking alternative e-cigarettes. Dr. Khan regularly publishes cancer papers in various peer-reviewed medical journals. He has been regularly invited to present lectures on various topics in complementary cancer therapy and pain and symptom management since 2000.

References

1. http://www.who.int/news-room/fact-heets/detail/cancer
2. https://www.ncbi.nlm.nih.gov/pubmed/2057036 A double-blind trial of a sixteen-hour transdermal nicotine patch in smoking cessation.
3. https://www.ncbi.nlm.nih.gov/pubmed/6434084 Placebo-controlled trial of nicotine chewing gum in general practice.
4. https://www.ncbi.nlm.nih.gov/pubmed/10053177 A controlled trial of sustained-release bupropion, a nicotine patch, or both for smoking cessation.
5. https://www.ncbi.nlm.nih.gov/pubmed/24029165 Electronic cigarettes for smoking cessation: a randomized controlled trial.
6. https://www.ncbi.nlm.nih.gov/pubmed/24830741 E-cigarette versus nicotine inhaler: comparing the perceptions and experiences of inhaled-nicotine devices.
7. http://canadianvapingassociation.org
8. http://ectaofcanada.com/
9. https://www.ncbi.nlm.nih.gov/pubmed/18377099 Use of Vitamin D in Clinical Practice.
10. https://www.ncbi.nlm.nih.gov/pubmed/27425218 Vitamin D and Chronic Diseases: the current state of the art.
11. https://www.ncbi.nlm.nih.gov/pubmed/26413186 Vitamin D and Inflammation.
12. https://www.ncbi.nlm.nih.gov/pubmed/16490556 Survival rates for breast cancers detected in a community-service screening-mammogram program.
13. https://www.ncbi.nlm.nih.gov/pubmed/19744825 Decreased accuracy in interpretation of community-based screening mammography for women with multiple clinical-risk factors.
14. https://www.ncbi.nlm.nih.gov/pubmed/23725113 Mechanics behind breast cancer prevention - focus on obesity, exercise and dietary fat.
15. https://www.ncbi.nlm.nih.gov/pubmed/20159820 Alberta physical activity and breast cancer prevention trial: sex hormone changes in a year-long exercise intervention among postmenopausal women.
16. https://www.ncbi.nlm.nih.gov/pubmed/20097433 Calorie restriction and cancer prevention: metabolic and molecular mechanisms.
17. https://www.ncbi.nlm.nih.gov/pubmed/25283328 Reduced signaling of PI3K-Akt and RAS-MAPK pathways is the key target for

weight-loss-induced cancer prevention by dietary calorie restriction and/or physical activity.

18. https://www.ncbi.nlm.nih.gov/pubmed/28841199 The Role of Red Meat and Flavonoid Consumption on Cancer Prevention: The Korean Cancer Screening Examination Cohort.

19. https://www.ncbi.nlm.nih.gov/pubmed/29185090 Meat consumption and pancreatic cancer risk among men and women in the Cancer Prevention Study-II Nutrition Cohort.

20. https://www.ncbi.nlm.nih.gov/pubmed/18592382 Dietary patterns and risk of bladder cancer: a factor analysis in Uruguay.

21. https://www.ncbi.nlm.nih.gov/pmc/articles/PMC1172224/ Eating meat more than ten times a week almost doubles chances of bowel cancer.

22. https://www.ncbi.nlm.nih.gov/pubmed/29910850 Role of gut microbiota in the pathogenesis of colorectal cancer; a review article.

23. https://www.ncbi.nlm.nih.gov/pubmed/29608253 The direct and indirect association of cervical microbiota with the risk of cervical intraepithelial neoplasia.

24. https://www.ncbi.nlm.nih.gov/pubmed/29317709 Increased Abundance of Clostridium and Fusobacterium in Gastric Microbiota of Patients with Gastric Cancer in Taiwan.

25. https://www.ncbi.nlm.nih.gov/pubmed/29181335 Perceived Workplace Stress Is Associated with an Increased Risk of Prostate Cancer before Age 65.

26. https://www.ncbi.nlm.nih.gov/pubmed/29021585 Perceived stress level and risk of cancer incidence in a Japanese population: the Japan Public Health Center (JPHC)-based Prospective Study.

27. https://www.ncbi.nlm.nih.gov/pubmed/15630849 The contribution of cytotoxic chemotherapy to five-year survival in adult malignancies.

28. https://www.ncbi.nlm.nih.gov/pubmed/26217661 Cancer as a mitochondrial metabolic disease.

29. https://www.ncbi.nlm.nih.gov/pubmed/24343361 Cancer as a metabolic disease: implications for novel therapeutics.

30. https://www.ncbi.nlm.nih.gov/pubmed/28250801 Press-pulse: a novel therapeutic strategy for the metabolic management of cancer.

31. https://www.ncbi.nlm.nih.gov/pmc/articles/PMC5554882/ Long-term stabilization of metastatic melanoma with sodium dichloroacetate.

32. https://www.ncbi.nlm.nih.gov/pubmed/27803917 Long-term stabilization of stage 4 colon cancer using sodium dichloroacetate therapy.

Chapter 10

Fasting: The Forgotten Cure

By: Ms. Josephine G. Marcellin,
MBA, PMP

Fasting has been practiced for centuries, in societies as ancient as the Greeks and in religions as old as Judaism. The purpose of these fasts varied. In the case of religious devotees, it was to engage in a deeper spiritual connection with God, or to practice the process of self-sacrifice, demonstrating that the mind and spirit were more powerful than the body. For other individuals, it was a method to rid the body of disease. By starving the body, it was found they could essentially heal themselves.

Jesus himself practiced fasting. In the Bible, it is said he went into the Judean desert for forty days and forty nights without food to pray and connect with God, to find inner strength and to prepare himself for his ministry, as he knew the path that awaited him would be rocky and terribly difficult.

So, what is fasting — and are the benefits simply mythical? Is there any science to back up the advantages so many have proclaimed?

Fasting is defined as "the willing abstinence [from] or reduction [of] some or all food, drink, or both, for a period of time." Simply put, it is creating an environment whereby the body no longer takes in external sustenance, but instead has an opportunity to regenerate. Fasting also provides the individual with the chance to build inner strength and allow them to regain power over their body and its material needs.

Fasting and Spirituality

Most religions, including Christianity, Islam, Baha'i Faith and Buddhism, practice fasting. Christians fast during the period of Lent, replicating Jesus Christ's sacrifice and withdrawal into the desert. This is also seen as an opportunity for self-reflection and preparation for the celebrations of Easter.

Muslims and followers of the Baha'i Faith also observe fasting from sunrise to sunset during spiritual periods. Lay Buddhists practice fasting during times of intensive meditation, such as during a retreat. During these periods, followers avoid eating animal products and processed foods. There is also a modified version of this fast called the "middle path." This method requires followers to eliminate eating after the noon meal in an effort to aid meditation and good health.

The Science of Fasting

Science has also illustrated the value of fasting. A recent study by Harvard researchers shows how fasting can increase lifespan, slow the rate of aging and improve health by altering the activity of mitochondrial networks inside our cells.

What are these mitochondrial networks? Mitochondria are like tiny power plants inside our cells. In 2016, a team of researchers led by Newcastle University demonstrated how mitochondria are fundamental to the aging of cells. Research from Harvard shows how the changing shapes of mitochondrial networks can affect longevity and lifespan and more importantly, how fasting manipulates those mitochondrial networks to keep them in a "youthful" state.

To demonstrate the effects of fasting on longevity, the scientists used nematode worms, which live for only two weeks. The study found fasting enhanced mitochondrial coordination and resulted in an increased lifespan for the worms.

Other studies also demonstrate the health benefits of fasting or time-limited consumption:

1. Dr. Satchidananda Panda, an expert on circadian rhythms and time-restricted feeding, found mice that eat within a limited amount of time (twelve hours) resulted in slimmer, healthier mice than those which ate the same number of calories in a larger window of time. This shows *when* one eats may be as important as *what* one eats.

The circadian clock, he found, even mediates the immune system. Mice missing a crucial circadian molecule had higher levels of inflammation in their bodies than other mice, suggesting conditions linked to inflammation, such as infections or cancer, may be positively affected by fasting.

2. Dr. Michelle Harvie, a researcher on diet and a specialist in calorie restriction and one of the first to demonstrate weight loss can reduce risk of breast cancer, focuses on what's called a 5:2, or two-day diet — a low-carbohydrate, calorie-restricted diet for two consecutive days each week. This model is sometimes called "intermittent energy restriction" or "intermittent fasting."

In her words, "People are eating constantly. They're not taking breaks from food — which I think is an issue." The 5:2 diet is a way to remind people they don't have to consume constantly. It can be done without limiting exercise (in fact, she highly recommends *continuing* exercise) and can encourage more balanced, healthy eating habits. Harvie recommends avoiding carbohydrates and focusing on proteins, which can help reduce hunger pains on the restricted-calorie days and on the normal days, maintaining healthy habits learned from the restricted days.

Her human studies showed benefits including weight loss and improvement in metabolic-disease risk markers. She is currently pursuing the connection between weight loss and chemotherapy, particularly how cells during a calorie-restricted diet may be better protected from the treatment's toxic side effects.

3.   Dr. Valter Longo, a fasting and longevity specialist, focuses on cellular health and periodic fasting. Periodic fasting requires limiting calories for between three and five days, such that cells deplete glycogen stores (glucose from food stored as energy) and begin ketogenesis (breaking down fatty acids for energy) — also known as entering into the ketosis state.

Ketosis is essentially a metabolic state in which the body relies primarily on fat for energy. Biologically, the human body is a very adaptable machine that can run on a variety of different fuels, but on a carb-heavy Western diet, the primary source of energy is glucose. If glucose is available, the body will use it first, since it's the quickest to metabolize. So, on the standard American diet, your metabolism will be primarily geared toward burning carbohydrates (glucose) for fuel.

In ketosis, it's just the opposite; the body primarily relies on ketones rather than on glucose. To understand how this works, it's important to know some organs in the body (especially the brain) require a base amount of glucose to keep functioning. If your brain doesn't get any glucose, you'll die. But this doesn't necessarily mean that you need glucose in your diet — your body is perfectly capable of meeting its glucose needs during an extended fast, a period of famine, or a long stretch of very minimal carbohydrate intake.

Dr. Longo employs the analogy of constructing a new building. First, you implode the existing structure and then you build the new one. "You destroy when you are starving and you rebuild when you refeed," he says. "Destruction is as important as the rebuilding."

To do this on a cellular level, cells must consume all existing glycogen stores and begin consuming ketones stored in fat, after the readily available glucose has been depleted. After three to five days of ketosis, you return to a normal range of calories again and the cells receive glucose to build back up, fresh and rejuvenated. "It's much more about the feeding than it is about the restriction," Longo says. "This combination can cause the destruction of damaged cells and replace them with functional ones."

What does this destruction and rebuilding lead to? In Longo's human study, published in February 2017, participants in his proprietary research experienced a significant improvement in body weight, waist circumference and BMI, absolute total body and trunk fat, as well as risk factors for aging and disease, including systolic blood pressure and insulin-like growth factor 1 (IGF-1).

In animal models, the results were even more profound. Subjects experienced extended longevity, lowered visceral fat, reduced cancer incidence, a rejuvenated immune system, improved cognitive performance and decreased risk factors/biomarkers for aging, diabetes and cardiovascular disease.

Dr. Longo also advocates Dr. Panda's time-restricted feeding as a good life practice, but suggests an intermittent energy restriction for only two days a week (the 5:2 diet) would not allow cells to enter into a fasting state. "The beginning of ketogenesis and the depletion of glycogen is the beginning of fasting," he says. And for that one must follow a guided low-calorie intake for at least three days, preferably supervised by a doctor.

Other benefits that have been cited from fasting include neuroprotection, increased insulin sensitivity, greater resistance to stress, endogenous hormone production and increased mental clarity.

How Do You Fast?

The answer to this question is really up to you. There are many ways to fast and as the evidence above demonstrates, there are multiple health benefits. So, the decision *to* fast is really the most important decision you can make

1. **Long fasts:** These, as demonstrated by Dr. Longo's results, are the most beneficial for weight loss and reduction of inflammation. However, all scientists highly recommend long fasts be done

under a doctor's supervision, especially if they extend beyond seven to ten days. There are many different types of long fasts:

    a. The most extreme is a "dry fast," consuming nothing at all (food or water). This is definitely not advisable, as it's very dangerous to go for more than a day or so without drinking.

    b. Water fasting means drinking only water and consuming no calories during the fast.

    c. During a combination fast, one drinks water only for seven days, then green juice for seven days and then blended green juice (including green apple or grapes) for seven days. It is called a combination fast as glucose is slowly introduced after the first week through the juice consumption.

2. **Intermittent fasting**: This is the more popular method of fasting, as it enables you to derive some of the benefits of fasting without going without food for an extended period. There are many forms, with the 16/8 being the most popular. 16/8 describes a sixteen-hour fast: fast for sixteen hours and eat only during the allotted eight-hour window, such as from 12 p.m. to 8 p.m. This process is a bit tricky, though, as the allotted fast time does not allow you to go into the state of ketosis—especially if you go back to eating whatever you want during your eating window.

When following a higher carb-based diet, once the fasting window ends, the body switches back to glucose-burning mode and bumps you out of ketosis (if you were in ketosis at all). If we go from eating a "normal" amount of carbs to shifting our carbs to very low, it can take at least two to three days for the body to even enter ketosis.

That means if you're eating whatever you want during the eight-hour window, you might not be giving your body enough time to get into ketosis at all.

To make this process work, you will need to adopt a ketogenic diet, which includes high fat intake, moderate protein intake and very low carbohydrate intake. This diet is designed to deplete your body of glucose (sugar) and trigger the breakdown of fat into ketones for energy. The ketogenic diet "starves" our body of glucose in the same way as fasting while allowing us to eat and provide our body essential nourishment.

You can also opt to modify the fast window from 16/8 to 20/4, or even do a full-day fast if possible.

My Experience with Fasting

In March 2016, I just couldn't get out of bed. Medical diagnosis revealed I was suffering from severe adrenal fatigue and chronic fatigue symptoms. My blood pressure was through the roof and my doctor wanted to put me on medication, but I resisted, believing there must be a more natural path to recovery. My research pointed to fasting as an option.

I decided to take the drastic step of going on a twenty-one-day liquid fast, but instead of simply doing a pure water fast, I opted to follow the combination method described above — seven days on water only, seven days on juiced greens and the final seven days on blended greens.

During the first four days, I experienced hunger pangs and severe headaches. I managed these by keeping myself fully hydrated at all times, going for nature walks and increasing my meditation and mindfulness practices.

By day five, all my hunger pangs were gone and I experienced a surge of energy quite unlike anything else I had ever encountered. I also noticed I was sleeping better. Over the next few weeks, I found I experienced a higher level of mental clarity and previously nagging joint pains had disappeared. My cravings also disappeared and I just had a tremendous improvement in my overall well-being.

At the end of my fast, I noticed a myriad of benefits:

- I had experienced not only a weight loss of eighteen pounds, but also had no cravings for processed foods, coffee, or sweets. My palate had definitely changed for the better.
- My digestive system also appeared to be working more efficiently.
- My sleep was a lot deeper and I woke refreshed every single morning.
- My joint pains had lessened dramatically and, in some cases, (like my left shoulder) had completely disappeared.
- My skin, nails and hair appeared more vibrant. My eyes were clear and radiant and I experienced much greater mental clarity than I had had in years.

For me, fasting was a definite lifesaver—so much so that I have made it an annual ritual, doing at least a five to 10 day fast every year.

What Happens When You Fast?

The most obvious benefit of these types of fasts is weight loss. If you're not eating anything, weight will drop off your body fairly quickly. During the first twenty-four to seventy-two hours, you go through all the glycogen in your liver. After that, your body needs to run on what it has stored, either protein or fat.

For the first few days, weight loss averages one to two pounds (.5 to .9 kilograms) a day, both because you're shedding water weight and because your body begins to change its focus from using ingested food for energy to using stored fat reserves for energy (ketosis). Since fat is more energy-dense per pound than protein, weight loss during this phase slows down to a more reasonable, but still rapid pace of a little over one pound every two days.

This makes for fairly easy weight loss, but fasting should never be used solely as a weight-loss method. It should be seen only as a side benefit. The real benefit is in getting your body back into balance to heal damaged cells, get rid of inflammation and really give yourself a reset button to turn on your energy and good health.

Your healing is the result of a process called "autophagy," which is like spring cleaning for your cells and is promoted by fasting. Since your body is essentially eating itself, it has a chance to get rid of any junk or waste material that may have built up and to repair the damage of oxidative stress. This is one of the biggest benefits of fasting, even for people who are already at a healthy weight, since it has powerful anti-aging and muscle-building properties.

One study also found an extended fast (ten days on average) was beneficial to patients with hypertension, also noting even though the patients didn't embark on the fast to lose weight, all of them did—the average weight loss was around fifteen pounds (6.8 kilograms). Longer term fasting (up to five days) may also have some benefits for chemotherapy patients.

137

Another benefit of extended fasting is purely mental: for many fasters, it's a way to reset their relationship with food, break free from patterns of emotional eating, or start fresh at the end of the fast.

Conclusion

Fasting is an effective method to aid and maintain weight loss, increase one's lifespan, reduce inflammation that causes cancer and other diseases, improve the body's capability to regenerate cells and get rid of waste, support more efficient energy production and usage and promote mental clarity and general well-being.

It is certainly not a miracle cure, but if you want to achieve optimal health, it is definitely one practice that should be adopted sooner rather than later.

As a transformation coach, one of the services I provide is nutrition and peak-performance counselling. If you truly care about your health and would like to live every day full of passion and joy, join our vibrant community by visiting my website, https://josephinemarcellin.com/leap.

You will:

- Learn the exact program I followed to have a successful fast, including the juices I made and the foods I ate when I broke my fast.
- Learn what I did to ensure there was minimal muscle loss during my fast.
- Receive weekly emailed updates sharing what has helped individuals like you take back their health and maintain high levels of energy consistently— simply by learning how to feed and nurture themselves

I hope to see you in the community. Until then, I wish you the very best of optimal health.

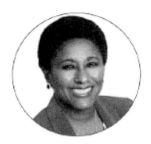

About
Ms. Josephine G. Marcellin, MBA, PMP

Ms. Josephine Marcellin, MBA, PMP is a formally trained Project Management and Finance Professional, with over 30 years' experience working in the Financial Services Industry. After working multiple 16-hour days and many seven-day weeks, Josephine fell victim to Adrenal Fatigue and required over 4 months of recuperation. During that recuperation period, Josephine made a commitment to completely transform her lifestyle in the same way she transformed her clients' businesses.

She became a raw vegan, incorporated mindfulness, yoga and increased movement in her daily practice, investigated ways to hack her sleep and gain greater depths of rest, as well as to fully understand the creation of an alkaline based ecosystem to fend off disease. Today, Josephine lives a joyful, healthy existence as a coach and mentor, helping others design a healthy balanced lifestyle that incorporates the principles she utilized to heal herself.

To learn more about Josephine, please connect with her:

Website: http://www.josephinemarcellin.com
Facebook:https://www.facebook.com/getresultswithjosephine/
LinkedIn: https://www.linkedin.com/in/josephinemarcellin/
Twitter: https://twitter.com/JosephineMarcel
YouTube: http://www.josephinemarcellin.tv/
Instagram: https://www.instagram.com/josephinemarcellin/
Pinterest: https://www.pinterest.com/jmarcellin/

139

Chapter 11

On the Road Again? Watch Out! The Business Traveller's Guide to Healthy Diet and Wellness

By: Mr. Charles Tchoreret

Looking back on my career, I am grateful for and at the same time humbled by the great opportunities I have had to travel to various countries around the world.

For twenty-five years I worked in the oil and gas industry as a professional supply-chain manager and SAP SCM consultant. My life was punctuated by regular business trips to various parts of the world. I worked in Gabon, Central Africa; in the Netherlands, Europe; in Nigeria, West Africa; and in Oman in the Middle East.

I also had the opportunity to travel to other countries, both for business and on personal account. I'm saying this not to brag, but simply to show, as I will explain further, how business travel can mess up your eating habits and as a result, your health and wellness.

The following includes an account of my personal experience as a frequent business traveller and testimonies from friends and colleagues who, just like me, wanted to get off this dead-end road.

My objective is to raise awareness of the dangers of a poor diet and sedentary lifestyle when you are on business trips. Being a business professional, be it as the owner of your own company or working for someone else, it is a blessing and I have no doubt everyone in that category has two main objectives:

1. To succeed in their business activities.
2. To remain successful for as long as possible.

Nobody wants to see their dreams cut short due to health issues, especially when it is the result of their own will.

I was there and I saw how my health was slowly, but surely going down the drain. I knew I had to take corrective actions immediately, before the self-destructive process became out of my control. I had to change my standards and adopt new rituals if I wanted to get myself out of this dead-end situation.

The way I felt about myself was my wake-up call. Unfortunately, most business travellers don't get that wake-up call until it's too late. They get caught up in the addictive life of easy access to food and drinks while they're on business trips.

The accumulation of bad eating habits, the way I felt in my own body and remarks from friends and family members on how I had gained weight brought me to the realization that something had to give—preferably not my health, but the poor diet and inactive lifestyle when I was travelling for business. I had to do something drastically different: maintain a healthy lifestyle away from home the best I could.

At home, I was fine. I ate a reasonably healthy diet and I exercised regularly. However, because of the frequent business trips, I found myself in a vicious circle. I was like a yo-yo: getting fit, then immediately losing my fitness in the span of a week's business travel. It was like starting from scratch all the time and my body did not like it at all.

Looking back to where it all started, I can describe the pattern with precision, as we will see later in the chapter.

The objective of this guide is to raise your awareness of the dangers surrounding your diet, coupled with the lack of physical exercise, when you're on business trips.

My Business Trip from Start to End

There is a perverse side to business travel that makes you lose focus on the level of self-control you must maintain at all times as far as your diet is concerned. Looking back to where I was, I can see exactly how I got "hooked."

My typical business travel started on week days with the alarm going off at 4 a.m. This was the latest I could wake up, since my flights were scheduled for 8 or 9 a.m. I had no other option. The booking was made by the company to ensure I arrived at my destination in time for the meeting, which usually started immediately after lunchtime the same day.

For every single one of my business trips, waking up in the morning was a struggle, I had difficulty sleeping every time I travelled. The night was usually very short and just when I started going deep into sleep, the alarm would go off and I'd literally have to drag myself out of Morpheus's arms. My stomach could not accept food so early in the morning, so I would head straight to the airport.

After a forty-five-minute commute to the airport and check-in, hunger would kick in as I headed to the business-class lounge to relax until departure time. Awaiting me would be well-presented displays of a wide variety of sandwiches, warm breakfasts, snacks, drinks and the inevitable aroma of fresh coffee.

Deep down I knew what would happen next . . . yet I justified my weakness by telling myself things like "It is not good to get on the plane with an empty stomach," "The flight might be delayed," "The food on the plane might not be as good as the food in the lounge," or "I can eat as much as I like for free!" Just a bunch of lame excuses to justify the unjustifiable.

As soon as I boarded the plane, located my business-class seat, stored my carry-on bag in the overhead compartment and sat down, more food and drinks would be offered.

During the flight, I'd try to catch up with my work before the upcoming meetings, take a quick nap or just do nothing. At this point I was no longer hungry, but still, the food kept coming. I could see it coming when I was awake and I could smell it when I was napping. There was no way out. Since I supposedly could no longer sleep, work, or relax and the food was there, what did I do? I grabbed something to eat.

During my week-long (or longer) work trips, the combination of sleep deprivation, business dinners and hotel buffets wreaked havoc on any plans to try to retain "at-home" meal routines.

All business travellers — without self-control—go through the challenges of self-destructive indulgence. Behind the glamour of free business-class travel lies the truth: a mess of unpredictable nutritional schedules and dietary temptations.

Consequently, even though I was health-conscious, I struggled to maintain a healthy lifestyle while travelling. Every business trip ended with me returning home feeling bloated, unhealthy and tired. Fortunately, I would take time to regroup between two trips, but before I knew it, the next business trip would be knocking on the door and the vicious circle would start all over again.

Know Your Weakness and Take Corrective Action

"Nothing is better than going home to family
and eating good food and relaxing." - Irina Shay

Watch out! Be on your guard against greed. Don't overindulge just because you have access to free food. It took me a long time to understand this and to apply this truth to my own life. After I realized how much damage I was doing to myself, I saw the analogy between the greedy wolf and the greedy business traveller.

Paul Harvey in The Rest of the Story series describes in vivid detail how an Eskimo kills a wolf. The process begins with the Eskimo coating a knife with animal blood and freezing it. He then adds another layer and another of blood, freezing each deposit until the blade is completely concealed. Next, the hunter fixes his knife in the ground with the blade up. After that, it is just a matter of time before a wolf, following his sensitive nose, finds his way to the source of the scent. He begins licking the blade and tasting the fresh-frozen blood. He licks faster, more and more vigorously, his tongue lapping at the blade until the keen edge becomes bare.

Feverishly now, harder and harder, the wolf licks the blade in the Arctic night. So great becomes his craving for blood, he doesn't notice the razor-sharp sting of the naked blade on his tongue, nor does he recognize the instant at which his insatiable thirst is being satisfied by his own warm blood. His carnivorous appetite just craves more and more, until the dawn finds him dead in the snow.

Business travellers may not collapse and die on the spot, but by repeating such behaviour they are putting themselves at risk for all sorts of health conditions that could lead to their perdition. They indulge in so much free food they forget they are their own judge, jury and executioner.

It Does Not Have to Be That Way

Once I became aware of the unfathomable abyss, I was letting myself sink into, I knew I had to do something about it. I finally accepted the fact that for every problem there is a solution. I stopped myself from being the victim of a situation beyond my control and pointing the finger at sources other than myself for the problem I was facing, I became a solution finder.

When you're willing to accept you're the problem, you immediately become the solution. I did not just take responsibility for success in my job; I also took responsibility for my inability to resist overindulging in food while on business trips. I had to acknowledge my own weakness and take control of my life. By accepting I was the problem and there was no bad fortune in play, my horizon of understanding opened up and I started seeing the course of action to take.

I realized for me to understand and overcome what I was going through and be in control, I had to change my focus through self-questioning.

1. How did I get there?
2. What went wrong?
3. What do I need to do to change the situation?
4. How can I break the pattern?

Finding answers to these questions was one good step forward. More importantly, however, I understood if I wanted to see lasting change in the situation and take control of my life, I needed to build some new rituals.

I knew the habits I followed were the result of rituals I had developed. We are controlled by our rituals more than by our intellect. Subconsciously, every time I travelled on a business, my focus was on the rituals and my anticipation of the trip. I was looking forward to the special treat I gave myself every time I travelled. I had developed a ritual that put me out of state, outside the normal behaviour I display when I'm at home.

I knew I had to go hard on this weakness to defeat it. What was amazing was not so much the end result, but rather, the satisfaction of seeing the change taking shape each step of the way. There was in me that sense of power over my weakness; I could feel it shrinking with every business trip I went on.

The only reason I got to this point is, as I said before, I started asking myself the right questions, targeted at understanding and assessing the situation to overcome it.

As a business traveller addicted to poor eating habits while on business trips, ask yourself these questions:

- What will I be proud of when I change this habit?
- What makes me proud right now as I tackle the problem?
- How do I breathe when I start feeling proud about foreseen success?

- How do I carry myself every time I find myself in the business lounge?
- What do I feel grateful about?
- How will I celebrate when I free myself from this addiction?

One thing to always remember: no matter what you want to change in your life, focus is controlled by questions. The quality of the questions you ask yourself will determine the kind of answers you get. Lousy questions produce lousy answers. Ask a better question and you will get a better answer.

For example, when you ask yourself "What can I do to maintain a good diet while on business trips," you open yourself to a range of solutions. Your brain is like a computer; you trigger the search and it comes up with an answer.

On the other end, let's say you ask yourself a lousy question like "How come I can't resist eating badly while on business trips?" The very fact you said, "I can't," tells your brain to come up with an answer: "You are a pig."

Deep down, you should ask yourself, *what does it really take to make that change?* Consider the old adage "If you want to take the island, burn the boats." When you burn the boats, there is no turning back; you have to find a way out of your situation.

What Does It Take to Successfully Make the Change?

From my own experience, I got to the point where I became sick and tired of my habit. I realized to kill that habit, I needed to have a more compelling vision of what I thought I wanted to do. I knew that approaching the problem without real determination would not be very inspiring for me, since I could not see what I would get at the end. It was like relying on my willpower to implement the change and I knew willpower does not last.

On the other end, having a clear vision of the new me, I wanted to create made me excited and I could not wait to see it materialize. I moved from pushing myself into making the change to being pulled by the vision of the new me. I could visualize myself walking into the business-class lounge and not being attracted by all the food on display. I could not wait to get to the next business trip to test myself.

As I will show you later, I did not just visualize. I took concrete action to back up my vision.

A Compelling Vision

My vision had to be something I knew would be gratifying when it was realized. Just saying what I wanted to achieve was not good enough. I had to raise my current standards so I could keep away from poor diet choices when I was travelling for business. It was a MUST. It was no longer a matter of "I should." My vision had these key characteristics:

- It was positive - I wanted my colleagues, my friends and my family to see the change.

- It was personal - I knew the satisfaction I would get out of it as far as my physical condition was concerned.

- It was possible - I had the "I can" attitude and I knew that my colleagues who were facing the same challenge would be interested to know how I made the shift.

- It was crystal clear - The clearer the picture of the change, the greater the chances of success.

Having been through this challenge, I know many other business travellers face the same situation. If this is the case for you, I want to work with you personally and help you through your own process. At the end of this chapter, you will find my contact details.

Preparation Is Essential

As I was going through my change process, I realized revising my standards meant adopting new habits. I had to prepare myself before every trip so my diet would remain as healthy as possible.

I started bringing my own snacks so I could avoid temptations from the unhealthy options at the airport food stores and in the business lounge. It worked pretty well. After two or three trips, I realized I was no longer attracted to what was on display and freely available to me. My snacks were more than enough. I always made sure to pack things like almonds and dried fruit and when I had to buy something on the go, I always went for healthy food.

Planning my trips in advance helped me a lot in the process. I wrote a list of all the snacks I needed, not just while in transit, but also on the plane. Various studies confirm airplane food, even in business class, is not nutritious and is loaded with calories. I also made sure to stay hydrated; water was all I drank. For those who like wine, it's alright to have a glass or two, but it is important to remain within your limits.

At the hotel and during business functions, I made sure to stick to my schedule. It is very tempting to eat the food people put in front of you. Earlier, I talked about raising your standards. If a scheduled lunch or dinner coincides with the time you normally eat, that's fine. However, avoid snacking in between, stick to your normal schedule and be content with what you ate. I know most conferences have a table in the back of the room with coffee and snacks for participants. If there's anything in the room you should avoid, it's any proximity to that table.

Also make sure you stay hydrated. It's fine to drink, but people should remember alcohol has calories and it dehydrates you. Again, always stay within your limits.

Eating Out

In everyday life, most of us probably don't eat out regularly. But on a business trip, dinners out are almost a daily occurrence, on top of bountiful lunches.

The temptation is to 'treat' yourself, especially when you don't pay for your own dinner. My advice: don't let yourself loose on the food. That's the worst move you could possibly make. When you are at home and you go to a restaurant, you make sure you don't overeat because you know doing so will affect your wallet. You normally go to a restaurant with friends and family to enjoy the meal, but also to enjoy each other's company and have a good time. It is not a competition of gluttony. Keep the same mindset during business functions.

If a big business meal is scheduled with your colleagues, eat lightly in the daytime, try to stick to one course and order extra vegetables or a green salad. If you have a dessert, have a non-creamy one or fruit.

Watch portion sizes in general, but especially if you are on business in the United States. I live in Canada and unfortunately, our portions are becoming more and more "Americanized."

You have the right to be assertive with waiters by specifying the quantity you want. You are the customer and they have to oblige. If you want your food cooked a certain way, or to substitute extra vegetables for fries, don't be afraid to say so.

One other major thing to avoid doing is feasting on bread. You know, that basket of garlic bread they bring while you are waiting for your order. I mentioned salad earlier, but ensure you order a low-calorie salad and a low-fat dressing like a vinaigrette.

Breakfast Time

This was another moment I could not resist. I know breakfast is the most important meal of the day, but I was overdoing it. I'm not advising you to skip breakfast. All I'm saying is buffets should be avoided.

If you want to keep satisfied all morning long—without the dreaded 10:30 a.m. hunger pangs—you need to make protein a big part of your meal. Foods like eggs and mushrooms are very good. Try to include some fruit and avoid sugar cereals. When you go for toast, go for wholegrain.

With a protein-rich breakfast you are less likely to snack frequently. I have never been a coffee drinker, but experts warn about going overboard at the espresso machine. You don't want to have more than three to five cups of tea or coffee a day. Don't rely on caffeine to keep you awake.

If you feel you are wilting, eat carbs instead of confectionery; it's much better to have a wholegrain sandwich than to grab a Mars or Kit Kat bar— the latter was my favourite. Chocolate bars are just a sugar hit. Unfortunately, sugar highs do not last very long and will leave you feeling drained afterward.

The Psychology of Eating

Back home, my family and I pray before every meal. Mealtime provides an opportunity to catch up with each other or simply to watch a tv program together. Eating alone in a hotel restaurant was something I could never get used to. It has always been hard to stomach.

In those moments of solitude, I'd find myself eating more than usual. I was compensating for the absence of my family. What encouraged me to indulge so easily was the fact the food was free. I could have as much as I wanted. For every bite I took, though, I felt excruciating guilt.

As I went through my change process, I had to find a substitute for my bad eating habits and eliminate the feeling of loneliness. The trick was to find an activity that would keep my mind off food. Physical exercise did it for me, as I will explain.

The shift helped me understand the psychology of overeating, a well-worn path a lot of business travellers go down. They feel lonely, they feel homesick, or they simply feel overwhelmed by the repetitive trips, so much so they compensate with excessive food and drink.

It's a scary place to be, looking at it in retrospect.

Add Physical Activity to Your Schedule

As we have seen so far, bad habits can creep in quickly when you're on business trips and over time they can have a serious impact on not only your health and well-being, but also your life in general.

Forget about going to the gym. From experience, I know after long work hours, going to the gym will not be your first priority. Make your hotel room your own mini-gym.

Fortunately, there are creative exercise options you can incorporate that go beyond the traditional hotel gym workout. You have to be creative and use what you have.

Tips that may be useful to you:

Start the day with exercise: Start looking for ways to slot physical activity for the first thing in the morning and add more before dinner, if time permits. You don't have to do all of everything; you can pick what you feel comfortable with. The key is to keep moving.

- Do cardio exercises.
- Run up and down the emergency stairs for five minutes.
- Do sets of burpees.
- **Strength building:** Use a chair in your room. Try one-legged squats (hold onto a wall or a table for support). Or, sitting in your chair, lift one leg up off the seat, extend it straight out, then lower and lift it for 10 repetitions.
- To work your chest, shoulders and arms, place both hands on your chair arms (make sure it's a steady chair without wheels). Slowly lift your butt off the seat (no pun intended). Lower yourself, but

stop short of touching the seat with your butt. Do 5 to 10 repetitions.

- **Work on your abs:** You can do a combination of sit-ups, leg raises, pulse-ups, plank crunches and side planks.
- **Build flexibility:** You can do neck rolls, shoulder rolls and quad or hamstring stretches.

There are, of course, many more exercises you can do. If you want to learn how to keep fit while you're on business trips, I'd love to work with you personally and help you on your journey to the new you. Be sure to refer to Divya's chapter for a female perspective on staying healthy while travelling.

Your Take-Away

We've established that behind the glamour of free business-class travel lies the truth: a mess of unpredictable nutritional schedules and dietary temptations. Even the most health-conscious business travellers struggle to maintain a healthy lifestyle while they're travelling.

I shared my personal testimony and how I overcame my addiction to a bad diet on business trips.

I shared with you why it is important to change your standards and start developing new rituals that will help you achieve your vision of the new you.

I am assuring you, you do not have to go through your transformation journey alone. It would be my pleasure to work personally with you and guide you through the process

Connect with me on Facebook and Linkedin "Charles Tchoreret",
Text me on 514-224-7012 or e-mail me ca@tcaconsultantsca.com

153

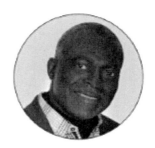

About
Mr. Charles Tchoreret

Mr. Charles Tchoreret is an experienced Supply Chain Management and SAP MM Consultant. He is a graduate of the University of Leicester in the UK, with an MBA in supply Chain Management and from the University of North London, UK, with a BA honour in Applied Language Study. Charles is a certified member of the Chartered Institute of Purchasing and Supply in the United Kingdom.

Before he retired in 2010, he worked for one of the largest oil companies in the world, where he held various management positions in procurement, contracts management and logistics. and travelled to over 25 different countries. As a leader in his church, he holds a weekly small group fellowship in his house. He loves sports and he is a keep fit addict. He is fully bilingual in French and English and has a good understanding of Spanish. As part of his sporting activities, he previously trained children and young adults, in Kyokushin Kai karate.
.

Chapter 12

Overcoming Adversity:

From Victim to Victorious

By: Ms. Hailey Patry

My heart longs for the day when all people who have been afflicted by adversity can stand proudly and tell the stories of their lives as victors, champions and heroes. Let's collectively release the victimhood and the blame many of us carry from our pasts. I long for the day when everyone can be grateful for what they have been through, that they have acquired the necessary learning and growth and that they have done more than just bounce back from their struggles—they have bounced better.

Before I share with you who I used to be, let me share with you who I am. To know me then is not to know me now. By the way, I am not sharing my story with you because my story matters. I am sharing it with you because your story matters and inside my story there is a lot of hope for the good that is coming soon from your story.

I am a mother, wife, sister, daughter, granddaughter, niece, friend, business owner, home owner, neighbour, provider, humanitarian and entrepreneur. Professionally, I am a speaker, facilitator, true-happiness and resiliency coach, consultant, marriage mentor, life guide, international best-selling author and offline success trainer. Personally, I am a lover, snuggler, giggler, romantic, dancer, kick boxer, traveller, adventurer, hiker, writer, poet and even a rapper when my eldest son invites me in for a rap battle. I am silly, funny, brave, bold, caring, strong, emotional and empathetic. I am also goofy, fun, successful, charitable, sentimental, deep, nerdy, quirky, social, outspoken, opinionated, committed, persistent, enthusiastic, driven and happy. Ironically, I am known as the "world's happiest woman," so what comes next might sound surprising.

I used to have no self-esteem, no self-worth. I body-shamed, was extremely depressed and suicidal and was a magnet for trauma.

I have lived through decades of abuse; eight years of anorexia and depression; two childhood suicide attempts; a violent rape; many surgeries; cancer; an unsafe first marriage; a tumultuous divorce, becoming a single mother at twenty-seven with a baby and six figures of debt; finding my soulmate and second husband, only to have our marriage tested in every way; fulfilling my dream of becoming a mother again then having my husband lose his job in the middle of my pregnancy; and like you, many other bumps and scrapes along the way. I have faced my mortality many times. Most recently, exactly a year before writing this chapter, I almost died from toxic shock syndrome, followed closely by a brain virus and months later had one of two surgeries to correct some other health challenges.

Today I stand proud as the champion of my life, a happily married mama of three miracle babies, at this time aged twelve, four and two. I stand proud to serve and inspire others and change lives every single day. Today I live with extreme happiness, love, joy and self-worth and it took something to get here. Everything I did is teachable and learnable and possible for anyone who has endured something hard and is committed to finding the blessing in it, doing the work to heal from it and continuing onward and upward.

I have been on many journeys within my overall journey to wellness and happiness, such as the journey to loving food, myself and life; the journey to cancer freedom; the journey out of depression and oppression; the journey to finding love (again and again and again); the journey to becoming debt-free after my first marriage ended; the journey to finally finding my soulmate; the journey to healing after our marriage was tested and wounded; the journey to conception through difficult pregnancies and home births; the journey to forgiveness and moving on; the journey through financial devastation and back to wholeness; and the journey to physical wellness through a variety of health challenges.

I once carried scars from all the battles of my life. I once and for a long time, felt deeply victimized, in endless victimhood, repetitive patterns and a non-stop onslaught of struggle.

Then everything changed. I will share just how later on in this chapter and even offer a complimentary coaching session as my gift to you, so that you too can access the perfect and timely methods to address what you are going through.

Today, I have no scars—all of the 'ugly' has become beautiful. I carry tremendous gratitude, extreme empathy for others and the ability to help others in a way that many cannot.

This is my wish for you, my reader, my friend: for you to feel as light, proud and grateful for your past and your story as I do about mine. For you to know it has shaped you or is in the process of shaping you into the very best version of yourself and to trust it had to happen to get you where you are now or where you are going. Which is something I call "You 2.0.
"It seems there is a very fine line between being victimized and victorious.

Access to crossing that necessary line comes through bridges such as forgiveness, empowerment, new learning, personal growth, choosing to pivot and take on a new path in life, making better choices, using negative experiences to inspire a new career, book, or view of yourself and so much more.

It also requires defining new standards, declaring new boundaries, clarifying what you want, 'uplevelling' your self-worth and self-esteem and healing your subconscious beliefs.

There are many natural and holistic approaches to healing from adversity and shifting your energy from victim to victorious. The best way I know is to share some of the events I experienced and share the bridges I used to cross over and become well again. So here goes. This is for you.

On a fall day in 1979, I was brought into the world by two loving parents who both had struggles of their own. Within their challenges, their marriage was rocky, too. They did the best they could for me and my two younger brothers, but amid their mental-health challenges, financial hardships and tumultuous relationship, my childhood was loud, often sad, unstable and challenging. At the same time, on the good days, they loved us to the moon and back and loved each other too. Today they are celebrating forty-five years of marriage and even though it has been tested and challenged, with age their personalities have softened and their love for us and for each other has grown. Everything they did wrong as parents they have more than made up for as grandparents to my three sons. Today, after forgiveness and healing, we are extremely close as a family. My parents call daily to see how we and the grandkids are doing and we see each other weekly.

My childhood left me with many scars, for many years. I was so confused by the rage coming at me, I interpreted it to mean I was not good enough, deficient. At the age of eight I believed I was worthless, disgusting and ugly. I began my eight-year battle with eating disorders and depression and fell into a deep, dark hole. The deepest point was when I was sixteen and tried twice in two weeks to take my life. I took approximately 600 pills, hoping to go to sleep and never wake up. It is for that reason and everything I put my liver through all those years ago, that I have never tried drugs or smoking and have never been drunk. I owe it to my liver to be nice to it forevermore.

The methods I used when I was sixteen to begin my healing journey included getting professional help, sharing my pain and my story with two trusted adults, journaling, writing poetry and writing out the balance sheet for my life. I also applied two strategies called The Gift of Perspective and Perpetrator's Compassion.

My encouragement to high school-aged youth is to speak to your guidance counsellor and special-resource team at your school. Don't suffer alone. There are caring and safe adults who can be there to listen and connect you with additional resources and supports to help you get through tough situations. I am also here for you!

The life-balance sheet is an exercise I did after surviving the second suicide attempt. I saw a counsellor who shared this very helpful tool with me. He encouraged me to literally draw a line down the centre of a blank page. In one column, I was to write all of the pain I could escape if I died and on the other, all of the future joys and accomplishments I would miss out on if I died. Doing that exercise proved to me that although my present challenges were massive and awful, if I chose to live there was so much waiting for me in the future: love, marriage, children, making a difference, helping others, leaving a legacy and so much more.

From this I learned the most important thing we all need when we are in a deep depression is a future to live into. We need a picture in our minds of a future potential life that has happiness in it, that seems worth living for. We all deserve the hope of a brighter future. And we need it!

From that strategy, I immediately realized I really wanted all of those things and it was time to stop focusing on everything that was broken in my life and start focusing on the future I wanted to create. I learned how to set, organize and plan for my goals. How to break them down into daily parts and stay committed to the life projects I was working on. I also learned that to have a brighter future, I had to work on myself, my self-worth and self-esteem.

I needed to let go of a lot of anger and resentment. At that time, I was not trained the way I am now. Today I am a master coach of Radical Forgiveness and Radical Living, teaching what I consider to be the world's best process for gaining closure, peace and freedom from the hurts, upsets, anger, blame, resentment and unforgiveness we carry.

As part of the healing process, I needed to see things from a different perspective. I had spent so long feeling sorry for myself. A few strategies helped that melt away. The Gift of Perspective allowed me to count my blessings. I pictured other young girls in different countries going through things much worse than I was and I would ask myself to be strong for them. I pictured some of what they were going through and knew that if they could get through their struggles, I could get through mine.

I also considered Perpetrator's Compassion in dissecting why the people who hurt me might be the way they were and the way they are. I knew it would not undo what they did to me, it would not make it okay and it would not condone their behaviour, but it certainly lightened the anger I had toward them and actually had me see both of us as victims, rather than just me. For example, when I think about my rapist from twenty-one years ago, I imagine he must have been through unspeakable things and also not be well in his mind, which turned him into the person who did what he did to me. I actually feel sorrier for him than I do for myself, because I have healed, I moved on, my life is wonderful, but if he is a broken man with a broken mind and no conscience, surely, he lives a miserable life and I feel badly for him.

When it comes to my attack . . . it came about a year after my suicide attempts. I was working on me, things were getting better, my confidence was returning, I was in a relationship and then it happened. My boyfriend at the time had been in a bad fight. Three men tried to steal his motorcycle and he beat them up very badly. He was a competitive fighter and advanced martial artist, so they didn't stand a chance. They decided to retaliate for how badly he had hurt them, there was no sense fighting him, as he alone was a lethal weapon, so they followed me for three weeks. Of course, I did not know any of this until after the attack, after I told my boyfriend about it and only then, did he come clean and tell me what had happened and who had done this to me. Thank goodness, it was only one of them!

One night in the spring of 1997, I was falling asleep doing my homework. You see, due to my parents' financial struggles, I had started working at a young age to make sure I ended up in a better place when I grew up. I worked two jobs every day after school and did homework into the middle of the night. As my head started to bob in fatigue, I figured I would go for a quick walk to get some fresh air and wake myself up. We lived in a very safe neighbourhood, so there was nothing to worry about.

He came at me from behind and took me down to the ground, weapon in hand. When it was over and I could feel the blood leaving my body, I knew a few things... This was both the worst night of my life in many ways and also how lucky I was to still have a pulse. Somehow it came to mind that others were attacked by more than one assailant and that others died on the ground they were left on.

Something changed inside me that night. A hero in me woke up. I required several reconstructive surgeries after the attack and it also caused cervical cancer, so I feel truly blessed to be alive and am thankful that although it was inhumanely horrid, it could have been so much worse.

While my body was healing, I worked hard to heal my mind, stop the nightmares and focus on bouncing back and bouncing better. I knew I needed to make a radical shift to move past this. I did not suffer in silence. I shared my story as part of a school project, coming clean about depression, abuse, suicide, eating disorders and rape and I encouraged others to come forward and share their stories so we could build a safe, supportive, non-judgmental community to heal together. Haphazardly I started my first group-coaching circle. By stepping into a support role, I had to make progress every day on my healing journey so I could motivate and inspire the others. That level of accountability really helped me make better choices than I otherwise would have.

One of the most important tools I developed and now teach, called 'Dreamcasting', is a nightly practice I highly recommend for any trauma survivors who get flashbacks, anyone with disturbed sleep and anyone who wants tomorrow to be brighter than yesterday. It is also exceptionally powerful for helping you to bring your dreams and goals to fruition.

I have a free thirty-minute voice-over presentation that explains the whole process and you can access it by reaching out to me and requesting it. All of my contact information is included at the end of the chapter.

When my body was strong again, I focused my attention on elevating my self-worth, taking my power back and raising my standards. I was still just a baby on that journey when I met my ex-husband. I still had a lot of work to do on me and since we choose our partners based on being a match for our self-worth at the time . . . I chose poorly. It was a very hard, loud and scary marriage. When I left for the safety of me and my child, my son was still a breastfeeding baby and I took on all of the debt my ex had. It was a very scary time in my life. I felt alone, unloved, financially broken and yet . . . I knew it had to be this way. There were lessons I still needed to learn and growth I had to go through. I dove head first into personal growth and quickly raised my bar. I was approaching thirty when I finally learned I am a 10!!! I am fully worth it, fully deserving, totally amazing and if I can love me, then a good man will too.

During the time before I met my husband, Jeremy (who as I write this has been my sweetheart for eight and a half years), I had a lot of work to do and many strategies to implement. Just a small bit of what I used to get strong and move on will be explained here. So, if you are someone who is currently in an unsafe relationship and need assistance creating a safety plan, game plan and personal care plan to get you out and get your life back on track, then please reach out. I am here to support you.

There is much more than what can fit on these pages, but here are some of the important steps I took that you can too:

1. I took on an additional income-generating opportunity so I could make more money to pay off the debt I inherited.
2. I worked closely with mentors and hung out in supportive environments to lift me up, such as personal-growth workshops and courses.
3. I asked for help from family and friends when I could not do everything on my own. Sanity is always more important than pride and people love to help if they are good people.
4. I became an amazing budgeter yet again and learned how to spend less, make more and eradicate my debt faster. I was forced into becoming more successful so I could provide for my son and myself.
5. I continued to work on me and make sure I was in the best shape of my life emotionally and physically.
6. I had a daily practice of affirmations and did my 'Dreamcasting' every night.
7. I used the same manifestation process I now teach all of my single clients to call love back into my life.
8. I was not afraid to share my story, to be open, to be vulnerable and lay it out on the line.

After these and other strategies, or bridges to cross over from victimized in a divorce to victorious as a proud single mama, I was ready to meet my soulmate and finally have it all.

After I became a debt-free single mom and my son was three, soon to be four, I was speaking all over Canada and the US sharing my story to teach others how they too could turn their lives around in all areas. Sometimes my audience had more than 20,000 people and sometimes my audiences were in banquet halls and living rooms. Eight and a half years ago, I gave a talk in Hamilton, Ontario and met the man of my dreams. I asked if anyone else in the room had children and no one did. I asked as a small joke if anyone wanted to borrow my three-year-old child for the weekend and he put his hand up from the back row and said, "Miss, if you're there, I will be there."

When Jeremy and I fell in love, it was epic. We dated for nine weeks from our two separate cities an hour and a half apart and then we bought our home in the middle. We were crazy and crazy in love. While we were building our life together, he also adopted my son, who is now our son. What a blessing it is for a little boy who is at odds with and has no contact with, his biological father to have a saint step up and raise him, love him and care for him. We are so grateful.

When our son was eight, we made his wish come true and gave him a baby brother. But there was a lot of struggle at that time. When I was three months pregnant, my husband made some big mistakes and lost his job and risked losing our marriage too. I was devastated half the time and over the moon to be expecting a little miracle the rest of the time. As you can imagine, it was a difficult pregnancy, but it led to the most magical and serene home water birth. The six months leading up to the birth were the hardest six months of my life, but this time I had all the tools at my disposal to heal, deal, bounce and thrive. And so, we did! But one tool was missing... Radical Forgiveness. I needed a new tool to truly move on from what had happened and that's when Radical Forgiveness came into my life. If you are still mad or sad at someone, or at yourself, I highly recommend looking into www.radicalforgiveness.com and the books, Radical Forgiveness or Radical Self Forgiveness, depending on whom you are upset with.

The other tools we used to heal our marriage and go from victim to victorious are the six steps I teach to my marriage clients on how to fall in love again and rewrite a marriage. In fact, I offer the basic steps as a free gift called "The Guide To Extraordinary Relationships," which you can access at the end of this chapter.

With the turn of events during that pregnancy, my husband became a stay-at-home dad and I later launched my full-time coaching institute, www.TheLiftedLid.com, to support my clients and to support our family. At the time of writing, my husband has been home for four and a half years; the strategies we used turned what was initially bad news into a huge blessing.

Because he lost his job, we learned to focus on what was most important and how to live on a lot less. We learned just how strong we are, how strong our marriage is, how forgiving my heart is, how caring his heart is and he learned he is truly loved unconditionally. When our middle son was eight months old, we excitedly began the pregnancy for our third son and nine months and two weeks later we welcomed our next miracle into the world. Now, as a family of five, we give our boys the rare and incredible opportunity to be raised by their daddy and have constant fun, adventures, excursions and male role modelling that so many children miss out on.

At first, the financial reality was crushing and it forced me to step up and learn how to help more people and earn more money. Because I opened up my hours and expanded my practice, I have prevented countless suicides, depression and divorces, helped countless clients find freedom from addiction, countless single clients find love, sexless couples to reconnect and fall in love with each other again, angry clients to find peace, frustrated clients to master themselves and their success goals. I am so thankful to have delivered happiness and resiliency training to thousands of students in 136 countries.

Trauma can be turned into triumph. Victims can become victorious. You can become the hero in your story and there are twenty-one 'Survive-and-Thrive' methods I would love to teach you and your loved ones, as well as your entire company and community, because happiness is teachable and learnable. So is the walk from victimhood to victorious.

Plus, it is absolutely worth it. Walking the path from victim to victor is worth every bit of gold waiting at the end of the rainbow after all of the storms. I want so badly for others to have what I now have. So much love, so much happiness, so much laughter, so much peace. I want this for you!

Today, I am so grateful that trauma and adversity chose me and allowed me to go through everything exactly as it did, so I could help the tens of thousands of people around the world, just like you, who now use my methods for their own healing, happiness and success.

Had I not experienced the violent rape, I would not be so effective with my clients who are also sexual-violence survivors. I love helping them feel safe, beautiful and empowered again in as little as one session.

Had I not experienced my own long battle with depression and suicide, I would not have the magical touch with my clients who are battling their own depression or suicidal feelings. I am deeply excited that my methods work in as little as one session to help children, adolescents and adults stop self-harming, stop considering suicide and start planning for happiness and joy in their lives.

Had I not been through an unsafe marriage, a horrific divorce and a very bumpy ride through single parenthood and financial ruin, I would not be able to support clients as lovingly, delicately and effectively through their own transitions of divorce, single parenthood and remarriage.

Had my husband and I not been tested the way we were, I could not be so raw and authentic while helping countless other couples to fall in love with each other again, as we too needed to go through the process.

You see, from today's vantage point looking back, everything happened exactly as it needed to and I am so grateful for having gone through it. At the same time, I would not want to go through it again, nor do I condone what was done to me or the choices of the people who hurt me.

But I do know this: my difficult childhood was perfect because it gave me the low self-worth and body-image issues that sent me into the fitness industry. Being in that industry was perfect because it is where I met my ex-husband and all of the awful things, he put me through were perfect because that marriage led to my incredible first-born son, all my ex's debt and the success story I became when I paid it off. Becoming that success story was necessary and working for nearly two and a half years to pay those debts off was perfect because it landed me on the speaking circuit which eventually had me talk in that room eight and a half years ago in Hamilton, which is where I met my Jeremy.

Meeting Jeremy and choosing him as my forever partner was perfect because he adopted my eldest son and helped me to create our younger two sons. All of the tests he brought into our marriage were also perfect because they have strengthened me, him and us; they have allowed him to be a stay-at-home daddy and that has allowed me to expand my coaching practice and serve, support and heal clients all over the world. I would not change a single thing. Based on how it has all worked out . . . all I can do is say "Thank you."

So, what is your story? How can I support you on your journey?

I am excited to offer you the gift of a complimentary coaching session so we can put a plan together for you to increase the amount of happiness, love and success in your life. Just as it was for the thousands of happy clients before you... You will come off the call feeling lighter, hopeful, excited and ready to implement some new actions into your immediate schedule to start shifting your circumstances right away. What are you waiting for, my friend? Today is a great day to claim your space in the world, turn up your light, fill yourself with love and have all the support you crave.

If you are truly ready to shine, then let's book you some time! You can text me on my confidential line at 1-416-797-5856 or email me at hailey@theliftedlid.com.

You can also request any of the available resources, such as the process for 'Dreamcasting', 'The Guide To Extraordinary Relationships' and most importantly, your complimentary one-hour session. Please send three potential dates and times, from 7 a.m. EST and onward and I will do my absolute best to fit you into my coaching calendar as soon as a spot becomes available. You matter. Your life matters. Your story matters. And I will make time for you because you, my friend, are amazing! Even if you do not fully see that yet.

From the bottom of my heart, I wish you love, joy, laughter, peace, vitality, abundance and to always know you are a 10!

With gratitude, love and smiles,

Your True-Happiness Coach, Marriage Mentor and Offline Success Trainer, xo Hailey

P.S. I would love to stay connected, keep in touch and add more love, endless laughter and abundant success to your life. Clients tell me that the results they could not get, after years of other therapy, they got with me in just a few hours. All of my amazing clients, people just like you, tell me they get immediate relief after our very first session. That's why I keep spreading the love!

Want to make your relationship EXTRAORDINARY? Get the FREE guide here: https://ws345-229b48.pages.infusionsoft.net/

I would love for you to add me as a friend on my personal Facebook page!

www.facebook.com/HaileyPatry
www.TheLiftedLid.com
ww.linkedin.com/in/hailey-patry-theliftedlid/

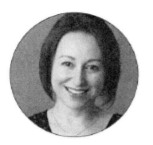

About
Ms. Hailey Patry

Ms. Hailey Patry is a 2-times #1 International Best-Selling Author, Coach, Speaker and Facilitator.

Hailey is a True Happiness Coach, Marriage Mentor and Offline Success Trainer. As a survivor and 'thriver' after more than 20 traumas, Hailey teaches you in a matter of hours how to triumph over adversity quickly and create your dream life both personally and professionally. She has been nicknamed "World's Happiest Woman" and she wants to help you achieve your happiest life. She has spoken for nearly one million people and supports 16,000 students in 136 countries. Hailey is the founder of The Lifted Lid, "Life Uncapped" and a Master Coach of Radical Living and Radical Forgiveness.

Hailey works with entrepreneurs, families, organizations and couples. In addition, Hailey is a seasoned business owner, having run a traditional business, an International franchise, a 60-million-dollar home-based business and a coaching institute. She mentors men and women to become the "2.0 version" of themselves, achieve their full potential, create successful relationships, a successful LIFE and a successful business/career. She is known for helping clients just like you, to achieve results in only nine session hours, that years of other therapies could not deliver. In fact, all clients report immediate relief after the very first session.

Chapter 13

Mental Muscle Fitness and Understanding Dementia

By: Ms. Maricel Gonzales

"Those with dementia are still people and they still have stories and they still have character and they are all individuals and they are all unique and they need to be interacted on a human level."
Carrey Mullingan

My Why on Dementia

I have always been interested in mental health, brain health, brain fitness and anything that has to do with the brain. My curiosity started when my grandfather was diagnosed with Parkinson's disease when he was seventy-eight. It took awhile for the whole family to notice he was suffering from Parkinson's — not until his hand tremors were more frequent and stronger. My parents had no clue, because he did not complain about anything and symptoms were very mild. His postural instability made his symptoms more evident. He started hunching over and moving slower than usual. His feet seemed to be stuck on the floor every time he walked and his body became rigid. He seemed to be very sad most of the time or have a masked face expression, like most PD sufferers. My grandfather went downhill because of complications from other medical conditions and due to his advancing Parkinson's.

This challenge in my family heightened my interest in mental fitness and human behaviour, particularly in relation to brain function and its complexities. Thus, human anatomy became my favourite subject when I was studying physical therapy. We studied the human brain from its physical appearance to the exciting point of opening a human skull, dissecting, studying its cross section and trying to memorize all its functions, innervations and composition. The brain is defined as one of the largest and most complex organs of the human body and it functions as the coordination centre of sensation, intellectual and nervous activity.

The reason I pursue my passion in writing about dementia is to share my knowledge, skills and personal encounters with patients living in the world of memory loss and share the psychological and behavioural changes that takes place as it progresses. I have also included some tips on how to prevent and delay the symptoms. My training in one of the biggest mental institutions in my country as a registered nurse made me realize this was the field I wanted to give service to. The skills I gained from handling different mental illnesses brought me to be qualified overseas and I handled the dementia unit, which we called the "locked-up" unit.

My understanding became deeper as I dealt with clients from different cultures, races, religion, values and beliefs, but nothing makes a difference when one is affected with dementia. What will make dementia exceptional is the type of care we render to patients and how we deal with them with love, care and compassion and by encouraging power and independence from their powerlessness and inability. Care is individualized and personal.

Caring for people with dementia is not easy, but it is more difficult for the client with all the changes that are unfamiliar to them. You have to have heart, passion and a ton of patience to provide the services they need. You feel their suffering, emptiness, longing for their love ones and sadness. You try filling the gaps between their thoughts and their missing words and you try to cheer them up and help them so they can have a quality and dignified life. The level of care depends on the type of dementia they have. Management is easier in the early stages on the caregiver's part, but acceptance is very difficult for the client and family.

Learning and understanding more about the brain changes and related issues will help in giving quality life and care for people with dementia to support them in preventing and delaying the progress of symptoms and help manage their condition with affection and power to go through life.

The rewarding part is seeing smiles on their faces. Don't dwell on the dementia disease. Focus on their strengths and abilities; value the moments; let them share their pearls of wisdom; let their smiles be more, laughter be louder and humour be a therapy. Get them involved in decision-making, promote independence and socialization. Keep them healthy and active and regularly connected with love ones. Do what is best for them. They are still human with so many stories to tell, lessons to share and a life to live.

Types of Dementia and Warning Signs

Dementia is the name for a group of disorders characterized by mental confusion, disorientation, memory problems, misperception and behavioural issues. It is caused by proteins that are toxic to the brain and damaged blood vessels and formation of plaques and tangles. The specific causes differ from one person to another, but a very common symptom is cognitive impairment or a decline in memory that leads to more complex personality change as it advances.

Symptoms affect memory, performance of activities of daily living and communication. There is a progressive decline of brain functioning or intellectual abilities.

Types of dementia are hard to diagnose in the early stages. Indications are often mistaken for normal signs of aging or side effects of medications and are usually underreported by family members or caregivers. The patient affected may not even recognize them or go to great lengths to conceal them because of embarrassment.

Alzheimer's Disease

The most common among all types of dementia. Forgetfulness is the most indicative symptom which is not a normal part of the aging process; however, increasing age is a risk factor. It usually occurs over the age of sixty-five, but early onset can occur under the age of fifty. Memory loss is the main concern with early onset. Forgetting names, telephone numbers, bank PIN codes, birthdays, or events that happened recently is one of the many things that define the characteristics of Alzheimer's disease. Carrying on a conversation, thinking and reasoning skills and completion of activities of daily living become a major problem as the disease worsens.

According to ilearncareerforce.org.nz, "as Alzheimer's disease progresses, abnormal proteins build up in some of the brain cells and these along with dead brain cells interfere with the nerve cells' ability to send and receive messages through the brain's network of neurons. Tangles, also known as neurofibrillary tangles, are formed out of dead and dying nerve cells called 'tau' protein, which bunch together and twist around each other to form tangles of nerve cell fibres (neurons)."

The Alzheimer's Association says, "these dead brain cells cause plaques and tangles to be formed throughout the brain. Plaques are deposits of a protein called beta amyloid that form around dead brain cells, as they form, they stick together into clumps (plaques). Plaques build up between nerve cells and prevent their ability to send messages to each other in the proper way."

Warning Signs and Symptoms
1. Memory loss that disrupts daily life
2. Challenges in planning or in solving problems
3. Difficulty completing tasks at work and leisure
4. Confusion with time or place

5. Trouble understanding images and spatial relationship
6. New problems with words, speaking, or writing
7. Misplacing things and losing the ability to retrace steps
8. Decrease in or poor judgement
9. Withdrawal from work or social activities

> *'The disease might hide the person underneath, but there's*
> *still a person in there who needs your love and attention."*
> Jamie Callandrielo

Gregg, husband of Roselyn, a seventy-nine-year-old resident in an advanced-dementia unit:

Gregg organized a fiftieth wedding anniversary with the help of the staff in the dementia care-lock-up unit. As the celebration started, Gregg stood by the door, well dressed in coat and tie, holding a bunch of white roses and a small paper bag.

One of the staff brought Roselyn from her room; she was wearing one of her special dresses.

As we settled her on a chair, Gregg walked to his wife, knelt on the floor, looking at her with teary eyes and uttered, "Happy fiftieth wedding anniversary, my love. I will always cherish the life and the days we shared together. If I have the chance to marry again, it is still you that I will choose. No other woman will make me a better man than I am today."

As we all watched, crying, Gregg brought out a small box from the paper bag. He opened it and said, "My love, take this ring as a sign of our life together. I will always love you forever."

Roselyn just quietly sat looking at Gregg with teary eyes the whole time during their renewal of vows.

Vascular or Multi-Infarct Dementia

According to the Mayo Clinic, "Dementia is a general term describing problems with *reasoning, planning, judgment,* memory and other thought processes. It is caused by brain damage from impaired blood flow to the brain"
https://www.mayoclinic.org/diseases-conditions/vascular-dementia/symptoms-causes.

It is the second most common type of dementia. It develops when the network of blood vessels, or the vascular system, that brings nutrients and oxygen to the brain is blocked. An interruption, blockage, or leak in this brain network is called a stroke. It can cause mild to severe damage to different parts of the brain. Brain cells eventually die if blood does not continuously flow to them.

Other medical condition such as an increase in blood pressure, high cholesterol levels, diabetes and smoking also narrows the blood vessels in cases of vascular dementia.

Edward, a forty-seven-year-old male, married with three children, working in research:

Edward had been experiencing headaches gradually increasing in frequency from once a week. He usually ignored or managed them with Advil. Once in a while he tried to exercise and get more sleep, thinking they were due to his workload and some family issues. He also tried to eat more vegetables, which he could not sustain because he is a meat lover and frozen, easy to cook food. After some inconsistent health management, he noticed his headaches were getting worse; to the point of not going away and having pain in his left eye. He became suspicious.

On his way home one day, he had a weird feeling. His hand could not make a tight fist and his right arm felt weak. He rushed towards home, but his arm suddenly dropped as he was driving. He pulled over on a side street and grabbed his phone. Worst of all, he was having a hard time finding his wife's number and calling 911 did not cross his mind.

He spent six weeks in the hospital and it took almost ten years of recovery for him to get back to his regular activities of daily living. Recovery was not 100 percent, but he continuously tried his best to reach optimum health day by day with the help and support of his medical team and loving family and friends.

Causes of Vascular Dementia
Stroke

A stroke occurs when there is a blockage or interruption of blood supply to the brain. This will result in oxygen deprivation, which will cause brain cells to die. Its' effects can be mild to severe, depending on the affected part of the brain. It is presented by weakness in the arms or legs, slurred speech, difficulty processing visual information and trouble with language and abstract thinking.

Narrowed or Damaged Brain Blood Vessels

Hypertension, atherosclerosis or build-up of plaques on the arteries and diabetes are some of the conditions that can narrow and damage blood vessels.

Signs and Symptoms may include:

Most common are problems with reflexes, difficulty concentrating and focusing, memory impairment, confusion, aphasia, urinary incontinence and retention, agnosia, difficulty performing goal-directed behaviour, depression, delusions, restlessness and agitation, difficulty in decision-making and inability to organize, plan and carry out a given task.

Parkinson's Disease

Parkinson's is "a progressive neurodegenerative disease. Movement is normally controlled by dopamine, a chemical that carries signals between the nerves in the brain. When cells that normally produce dopamine die, the symptoms of Parkinson's appear"
http://www.parkinson.ca/about-parkinsons/understanding-parkinsons/.

The Natural Institute of Aging (NIA) defines Parkinson's as "a brain disorder that leads to shaking, stiffness and difficulty with walking, balance and coordination."

> *"I often say now I don t have any choice whether or not I have Parkinson s, but surrounding that non-choice is a million other choices that I can make."*
> *Michael J. Fox*

Fifty percent more men than women are affected. It usually occurs around age sixty, but in some studies 5 to 10 percent experience early onset—before the age of fifty. Parkinson's disease results from a combination of genetic factors that make it hereditary. Exposure to toxins and other environmental factors and genetic mutations can cause it to occur randomly.

Signs and Symptoms may include:

Common symptoms include depression, mental problems, difficulty walking and talking, hand tremors, or shaking and pill rolling, bradykinesia, muscle rigidity, impaired posture and balance, Parkinsonian gait (leaning forward and taking small, quick steps); decrease in performing unconscious movement; monotone speech, difficulty writing and incontinence and constipation.

Lewy Body Dementia

The hallmark brain abnormalities linked to LBD are named after Frederich H. Lewy, MD, the neurologist who discovered them while working in Dr. Alois Alzheimer's laboratory during the early 1900s. It is a common form of dementia, but often misdiagnosed. Its' symptoms are a combination of Alzheimer's and Parkinson's disease. It is caused by abnormal deposits of a protein called alpha-synuclein. These deposits deplete dopamine, a neurotransmitter located in the brain stem. When the protein reaches other parts of the brain, it affects more brain chemicals, such as acetylcholine, located in the cerebral cortex. This part of the brain is responsible for behaviour, perception, decision-making and thinking.

LBD has no cure. The array of presenting symptoms from Parkinson's and Alzheimer's disease makes it more difficult to manage. The medication carbidopa-levodopa for Parkinson's will manage muscle rigidity. Sleep, memory and cognitive function can be managed with rivastigmine, which increases the neurotransmitters of the brain. These medications have side effects that have to be managed.

Signs and Symptoms may include:

Loss of motivation and planning, confusion, changes in reasoning, extreme fatigue, hand tremors, feet and limb spasms, apathy, depression, hallucinations, delusions, difficulty sleeping, drowsiness, blank stares, decreased attention span, disorganized speech, memory loss, cognitive problems, disrupted automatic body movements, constipation, anxiety and an impaired sense of smell.

Helpful Therapies

Listening to soothing music can manage anxiety and frustration. Aromatherapy can help mood and behaviour. Massage therapy, exercise, pet/animal therapy and cognitive and behavioural therapy have also been helpful.

Robin Williams, an American actor/comedian, died by hanging himself at age sixty-three. Some of his famous movies are Dead Poets Society, Awakening, World's Greatest Dad, Aladdin and Good Will Hunting.

According to *Scientific American,* "In the months before his death, Robin Williams was besieged by paranoia and so confused he couldn't remember his lines while filming a movie, as his brain was ambushed by what doctors later identified as an unusually severe case of Lewy body dementia" (https://www.scientificamerican.com/article/how-lewy-body-dementia-gripped-robin-williams1).

Susan Scheider Williams, wife of Robin Williams:
"As you may know, my husband Robin Williams had the little-known, but deadly Lewy body disease (LBD). He died from suicide in 2014 at the end of an intense, confusing and relatively swift persecution at the hand of this disease's symptoms and pathology. He was not alone in his traumatic experience with this neurologic disease. As you may know, almost 1.5 million nationwide are suffering similarly right now" (Neurology Journal, September27, 2016).

Fronto-Temporal Dementia (FTD), or Pick's Disease

Fronto-temporal dementia, formerly known as Pick's disease is a group of related disorders that affect the frontal and temporal parts of the brain. It is irreversible and progressive. The nerve cells shrink and deteriorate. Onset range from forty-five to sixty-five years old, according to the Alzheimer's Association. No prevention or cure is available and the disease progresses steadily.

It is hereditary. It is commonly misdiagnosed as addiction, Parkinson's disease, bipolar disorder and schizophrenia. No medication or treatment is available to delay the progress of this devastating disease. The life span once this dreadful disease is diagnosed ranges from two years to ten years as per theaftd.org

Anti-psychotics and anti-depressants are the drugs of choice to manage the symptoms of behavioural problems. Intervention and building alternative ways to communicate can be achieved with speech therapy. A comfortable environment away from crowds is ideal for people with FTD.

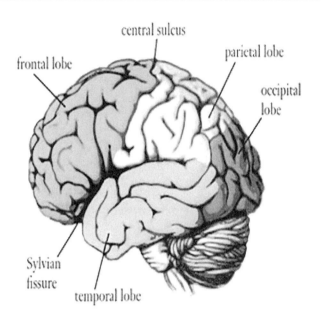

Symptoms include:

Socially inappropriate behaviour	Loss of memory
Focus on repetitive or compulsive routines	Lack of inhibition or restraint
Difficulty understanding words and naming objects	Lack of empathy
Neglect of personal hygiene and care	Apathy and depression
Loss of reading and writing skills	Clumsiness and frequent falls
Difficulty thinking and concentrating	Stiffness and slowness of movements
Problems with reasoning and judgement	Difficulty speaking and understanding

Variant Creutzfeldt-Jakob disease (CJD

Variant Creutzfeldt-Jakob disease (CJD) is a "relatively new and rare neurological disease, classified as a transmissible spongiform encephalopathy (TSE). It was first identified in March 1996 in the UK, when ten cases of a new disease with neurological symptoms were reported and soon associated with the Bovine Spongiform Encephalopathy (BSE), 'mad cow' disease." (European Centre for Disease Control)

It is characterized by a fatal neuronal degeneration through the formation of tiny holes in the brain. Brain cells are eventually destroyed due to the formation and accumulation of infectious and abnormal prion proteins. A cure has not been found and the condition is fatal. Symptoms are similar to Alzheimer's and Huntington's disease.

According to https://www.ninds.nih.gov/Disorders/Patient-Caregiver-Education/Fact-Sheets/Creutzfeldt-Jakob-Disease-Fact-Sheet, "the onset of symptoms occurs at about age 60 and about 70 percent of individuals die within one year." It affects one person in every million annually. It is hereditary, sporadic and acquired. Rapid progression to dementia is one of its hallmarks. Spasmodic and myoclonic involuntary movement of muscle groups follows.

Symptoms evolve over days and weeks rather than over years and typically include personality changes, mood and behaviour changes, memory loss, anxiety, depression, impaired thinking, worsening myoclonus, blindness, impaired judgement, insomnia, difficulty speaking and swallowing, sudden, jerky movements and coma.

Tips on Preventing Memory Loss
- **Brain and Memory Booster Food**

Brain food matters for our grey matter. What we eat is what we are. The link between our nutrition and mental function says a lot about our health.

Brain Foods Include:

Fish (wild salmon), garlic, coffee, avocado, blueberries, broccoli, spinach, kale and other leafy greens, coconut oil, olive oil, beans, turmeric, pumpkin seeds, dark chocolate, nuts, oranges, eggs, green tea, red wine, cayenne pepper, kimchi, rosemary, beets and fruits.

- **Vitamins for Mind Power**

Vitamins and nutrients have always been recommended as supplements to enhance our overall health and boost memory power. They also help to stimulate or activate some chemical agents that are important for the brain-memory function. There's a link between brain power and vitamins. They help carry oxygen to the brain. Some of those listed below will help you gain better mood, sharper memory and better attention span.

Vitamins for Mind Power Include:

Vitamin B complex: B1 (thiamine), B2 (riboflavin), B3 (niacin), B6 (pyrodoxine), B12 (cyanocobalamin), choline, vitamin C, vitamin D, CoQ10, vitamin E, Gingko biloba, carcumin from turmeric, fish oil, omega fatty acid, acetyl-L-carnitine, DHA supplements, phosphatidylserine supplements, Bacopa monniere, antioxidants, beta-carotenes, Gotukola and Rhodiolarosea.

- **Daily Habits for Mental Fitness**

Maintaining our mental health is just as important as taking care of our physical fitness. Having a daily or regular routine keeps our life in balance and in harmony with productivity and longevity. Keep yourself moving. Just move. Do anything as long as you don't stay in one place. If you get stuck in your emotions, you end up having maladaptive thinking.

- **Healthy Daily Routine Tips**

Exercise, dance, listen to music, practice belly breathing, eat a balanced diet, connect with social groups, express gratitude, spend time outside, meditate, have a good laugh, do deep-breathing exercises, sing, get good sleep, have something to look forward to, try to learn new things, reach out and hug someone, go places, read, solve crosswords and puzzles, play board games, relax, relax, relax, go to the beach, etc.

Handy Wisdom to Live By

"My secret to reaching my age is no secret. Just keep going and don't stop, just don't stop. Try to push yourself even if you feel lazy. Keep your body and brain healthy by eating healthy and moving, that's the only way to live my age." - Harry Katz

Harry Katz, an active, witty, ninety-seven-year-old male client:

Harry, being the youngest and the only boy in his family with five sisters, said he had a happy, active and enjoyable childhood. He used to be a runner and exercised regularly. His late wife, Marjorie, is very active in sports as a professional swimmer. His children are also active in different sports and arts, an interest they acquired from both parents.

At ninety-seven, he regularly wants to have breakfast at McDonalds, which he had been doing for eight years. He would always order his blueberry muffin and coffee and share a table with his regular breakfast buddy. He loves a spoonful of coconut and olive oil daily and his lemon water to keep him hydrated. Hypertension is one of the few medical concerns he has, but it is well managed.

He likes to do "mini-walks" after breakfast and go to the gym for an hour of stretching and biking. He takes a nap when he goes back home and his lunch is always around 2 p.m. and dinner at 6 p.m., which includes soup, his undying chicken teriyaki and vegetables.

Daniel, his son takes him to their favourite hang-out area, the Kensington Market every summer for ice cream treats. Yonge and Bloor street is a favourite walk night destination when the weather is good.

He loves to read books, journals, magazines and newspapers and do his crossword puzzle. He keeps a journal of his ADLs. He watches his favourite comedy duo, Wayne and Shuster shows on YouTube and his news on TV. He regularly walks for about forty-five minutes a day in the afternoon while he listens and sings along with his energizer song, "Top of the World" by Karen Carpenter, with his own never-ending lyrics, "di,di,di,di." He has a very good sense of humour and enjoys good conversation.

PSW: Mr. Katz, did you go to Baycrest today?
Mr. Katz: Yes, but I did not enjoy the lunch.
PSW: Why, what happened?
Mr. Katz: The people I sat with at lunch are all quiet. They don't talk, thats why they grow old.

(Mr. Katz is the oldest and bubbliest among the clients that sit with him in the dining hall.)

"A lack of social stimulation is harmful for people living with dementia. It exaggerates the impact of the condition that can lead to depression and it encourages the person to withdraw into themselves." - The more you keep your thoughts, feelings and actions focused on your target goal, the more likely you will get to achieve your goal.
Bob de Marco, AlzheimersReadingRoom.com

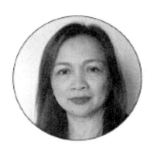

About
Ms. Maricel Gonazles

Ms. Maricel Gonzales, a happy person with tons of high energy and a good soul. Her personality connects her so strongly with the people around her and to the people she works for. She is very passionate about making a difference and sharing her knowledge in elder care and mental health challenges.

Maricel's humanitarian qualities, nursing background, physical therapy studies, extensive trainings and working in hospitals, mental institutions and big nursing homes in the Philippines and New Zealand, especially in advance dementia unit gave her a broad base on her approach for her chapter. Migrating to Canada gave her passion more life and meaning that fuelled it to be on fire.

Chapter 14

Release, Let Go and Do Yoga

By: Ms. Tiffanie Carr

Yesterday I was clever,
so I wanted to change the world.
Today I am wise, so I am changing myself."
Rumi

My Life Pre-Yoga

We all have them: moments in life when we feel change coming. It could be a decision we make, an opportunity we accept, or a multitude of other things that create different paths for us to take on this road we call life. In my case, I'll share two specific defining moments that changed my course.

It started when I was a child. I was three years old when my mom realized I had trouble speaking. After countless therapist visits, it was concluded that I had a serious speech impediment that caused me to utter sounds that nobody could understand. This condition also affected my ability to learn.

Fortunately, today I'm a chatterbox, but back then, it was painful because I had trouble connecting with people, especially kids. However, what affected me the most was the bullying. Some kids were mean and said hurtful things. The bullying got worse when I had to retake a year in school. As a result, I became anxious and didn't like school. I remember frequently writing "I HATE LIFE" in my school books.

My first defining moment came on the worst day of my young life. It was my best friend's graduation day (what would have been my graduation) and I was to be her guest. As I biked to school, I was excited to see her, but when I arrived in the front yard, my bullies were there, amid a sea of kids wearing their graduation gowns, shouting, "What are you doing here? You don't belong here, you're soooo stupid." They kept yelling cruel, awful things as I kept riding off the school property and as far away as I could get from them. That day I cried until I had nothing left to cry. I decided things needed to change and they did.

The following years I worked harder than ever with speech therapists to overcome my speech and learning challenges. Gradually, my grades went up and my communication skills improved. I even graduated high school with honours in history. Although on the outside things looked great, on the inside they weren't. I still felt like "that stupid little girl". This feeling followed me throughout my twenties and into my thirties. I was depressed and some days, I had trouble getting out of bed.

189

Can you relate to any of this? If you can, then you may know the feelings of hopelessness that come with depression. The good news is that there is hope and, in my case, it came in the form of yoga, my second defining moment.

One day, a friend was telling me how much joy yoga brought to her life. She went on about the benefits of practicing yoga and how it kept her calm and happy and helped her cope with mood disorders. I was sold. My local gym offered yoga and I began classes immediately. I craved for the same positive feelings, my friend experienced with her practice, but I never expected how life-changing it would be for me.

After each class, I came home feeling better about myself. I lost weight, felt confident and energetic, slept better and I was able to refocus my energy on my breath when things around me were stressful. I felt a renewed sense of self as yoga brought inner peace and balance back into my life.

My friends and colleagues started commenting on my posture and noticed I looked happier. I was! I was even smiling more. After about a year and a half of practicing yoga, my instructor was planning a big move across the country and recommended me as her replacement. That opportunity showed up during the period when my journey into the world of yoga deepened as I worked toward becoming a certified yoga instructor.

Just as yoga helped me forgive my bullies and heal an old wound from my past life, I was also able to help others. After all, we all have stories from our past whose villains need forgiving and through mindful meditation, visualization and a regular yoga practice, we can release and let go of pain. As a good friend once said, "Yoga is a journey of the self, through the self, to the self."

Although most people do yoga hoping to release tight muscles, get fit and perhaps feel less stress, my goal today is to share how it can help you reconnect to yourself on a much deeper soul level. For the majority of people, that's where there's usually a disconnect. Today, allow yourself to open your heart to the gift that is yoga. You couldn't be in a better place than you are right now.

What is Yoga?

What comes to your mind when you think about yoga? Fitness? Flexibility? Breathing? Lululemon? When it comes down to it, yoga is a very broad subject and can mean a multitude of things to different people. For me, yoga means freedom. Freedom from stress and fear and freedom to just be. In yoga, it's just me and my mat.

The textbook definition of yoga is the union of breath, body and mind. In fact, the Sanskrit root of yoga is "yuj" (which sounds like "yugh"), and means to unite and/or to control.

In this chapter, my goal is to focus on how yoga can serve you and improve your quality of life. We will journey into vital yoga postures (asanas) that will help you release tension in your body to help you feel your best, breathing exercises (pranayama) to help you feel calmer and more alert and meditation practices for a peaceful mind, body and soul.

One last word: you don't need to be experienced to benefit from yoga as it can be personalized for anyone, from beginners to more advanced learners. Be sure to check with your healthcare professional if you have any medical condition.

What You'll Need to Practice Yoga
The good news is that yoga is an activity that requires very little to no equipment at all. Typically, the minimum is a yoga mat, but keep in mind that a towel or blanket on a carpeted floor would do just as well.

If you're practicing indoors, make sure you're in a warm, open space. If you feel like you might need additional props, like blocks, straps, blankets, or bolsters, those can be purchased online or at your nearest discount department stores.

As for what to wear, keep it simple, stretchy and comfortable. Many yogis prefer clothes that can move with them from pose to pose.

Asanas
Moving your body is essential in creating more energy and vitality in your life. It's with movement that we feel better about ourselves. We can even turn a bad mood into a good one simply by stretching, shaking and moving our bodies. Without movement, our bodies feel sluggish, tense and heavy (the term "couch potato" comes to mind).

A great way to get your body moving and feeling incredible is to practice yoga poses, also known as asanas. Although many people make the mistake of thinking that getting adequate physical exercise requires high-intensity activities, the good news is that increasing your heart rate is doable through the practice of asanas (yoga poses performed in sequences). Asanas are the trademark of yoga. These poses help in improving your overall flexibility, strength and well-being. Asanas are performed at a slower pace with controlled movements, stretches and deep breathing, which also helps avoid lactic acid buildup.

For this next portion, we'll be looking at two powerful sequences that can be incorporated into your morning routine or at night before bedtime. As an added bonus, I'll include five other sequences that can be practiced at any time and will be suitable for any level of yoga practitioner. These are offered to you on my website, TiffanieCarr.com, under the tab "Yoga Sequences." Log on anytime through your smartphone or laptop and let me guide you through sequences that will make you feel rejuvenated.

The following sequences are in the tradition of Hatha yoga, which means sun (ha) and moon (tha) in Sanskrit.

Hatha yoga's purpose is to:

"unite and balance the solar (energizing) and lunar (relaxing) energies of the body"
Kristie Dahlia, The Body Shop Yoga

Morning Sequence

For this morning sequence, I recommend setting your alarm thirty minutes before your usual wake-up time and making this part of your self-care routine. This sequence will begin the moment you wake up in bed and find your way to your mat.

Lying in bed with your eyes closed, begin waking up with three deep breaths (read more on breathing in the next section). Your goal right now is to reconnect to your body, breath and soul and to achieve this, set an intention on how you wish to feel. For instance, you may want to feel less stressed today than you were yesterday. What might you need to do to accomplish this?

As you set your intentions, begin to slowly add gentle movements. Start by wiggling your toes, then rotating your shoulders and ankles for 1 - 2 sets of 5 repetitions, followed by opening your eyes and mouth wide and then closing them for 5 repetitions. Completing your rounds, slide out of bed, unroll your mat and get ready for your morning sequence.

Sun-Warrior Standing Poses

Standing poses offer a mind-body awareness and will help you release any tightness caused by sleep-related muscle stiffness or stress. These poses will also help strengthen your posture so you feel in alignment for your day ahead. Allow yourself the freedom to modify and tweak these poses for your body, fitness level and strength. Note: Hold poses for 3 to 5 deep breaths and increase as you keep going.

1. Mountain pose (tadasana):

Standing at the top of your mat, find equilibrium by placing your feet hip-width apart. Let your arms loosen by your side with palms facing your thighs. Ensure your feet are anchored into the ground with your weight evenly distributed. Feel your energy move from your lower body all the way up to the crown of your head. Lift your sternum up and soften your shoulders away from your ears.

2. Crescent moon pose (ardha chandrasana):

From mountain pose, inhale and lift your arms over your head and interlace your fingers. Feel your body lengthen from both sides while your shoulders soften down away from your ears. Exhale and bend sideways from the waist to the right. As you hold the pose, make sure to keep a long neck and move the crown of your head slightly toward your hands. Repeat on the left side. If at any time you feel tension in your lower back, either widen your stance or perform this pose seated on a block on the floor. As you return to centre, bring your hands back down alongside your body into mountain pose.

3. Standing camel (ustrasana):

From mountain, slide your hands on your lower back, above your hips, with your elbows bent 90 degrees. Inhale and move your shoulder blades closer together as you lift your sternum upward. Lift your chin slightly, but don't drop your head. Engage the muscles of your buttocks and hold for fifteen to thirty seconds. Then slowly start releasing your pose and return to mountain pose.

4. Chair pose (utkatasana):

Inhale and lift your arms overhead with palms facing each other. As you exhale, squat down, bending your knees 90 degrees. Drop your tailbone down to protect your lower back from arching, root your heels into the ground and look forward. For a refreshing twist to this pose, add pulsing by lowering and raising your hips one inch for 10 to 20 repetitions. Then, stand back up into mountain pose.

5. Warrior II (virabhadrasana II):

This pose is one my favourites, as it represents power and focus while it strengthens your arms and legs. To move into this from the mountain, take a step back with your left foot (about one leg-length) toward the rear of your mat. Your left foot turns out at a 45-degree angle with your toes pointing towards the front of the mat and your left heel aligned with your right heel. Bend your right knee at a 90-degree angle so your right knee is over your right ankle. Ensure that your torso is above your pelvis, then turn your torso towards the left side of your mat. Lift your arms at shoulder height with your right arm directly above (and parallel to) your right thigh. Your arms should be strong as they hold still. Move on to the next pose (#6) before repeating this pose on the left side).

6. Reverse warrior (viparita virabhadrasana):

From warrior II, with your right knee bent above your right ankle, begin to lift and rotate your right wrist over your head as you lower your left hand gently down on your left leg. Relax your shoulders and lift your chest up. Let your tailbone drop to avoid any pinching in your lower back. Gaze up at your right hand and hold for 3 breaths. Return to mountain pose and repeat warrior II and reverse warrior on the left side.

7. Standing forward fold (uttanasana):

From mountain, inhale and lift your arms overhead. As you exhale, dive down toward the ground by hinging at the hips and bending your knees slightly. Bring your forehead closer to your legs and touch the floor with your fingertips or use blocks for support. Feel your spine lengthening as you bring your head down toward the floor and lift your hips up. Allow your upper body to release into this pose. Benefits: This pose is great for your nervous, endocrine and digestive systems. Then, lift back up into standing in mountain pose.

End this morning sequence with 5 deep calming breaths and if time permits, redo this sequence 2 or 3 times, adding more time with each hold. Make sure to log on to TiffanieCarr.com for more sequences.

Night Sequence

As you settle down after a long day, it's vital to reconnect with yourself and release any strain and anxiety that may be lingering in your body. Instead of passing out on the sofa in front of the latest Netflix show, opt for the following poses to help relieve lower back strain, open tight hips and return to harmony: the perfect medicine for a good night's sleep.

Bedtime Yoga Poses

For this sequence, make sure you're ready for bed, meaning your face is washed and teeth are brushed. Have soft music playing in the background and wear comfy clothes or your pyjamas. Try using essential oils (I like combining vetiver and lavender as they help relax the mind and promote restful sleep) and then gently begin this practice. **Note:** Hold for 5 - 10 deep breaths on each side.

1. Easy pose (sukhasana):

This is a crossed-legged pose. From a seated position on your mat, cross your legs and flex your feet into a comfy pose. If you feel any tension in your lower back, sit on one or two folded towels or blankets and ensure that your knees rest below your hips. Feel your spine lengthen as you lift the crown of your head upward. From there, raise your arms over head, interlace your fingers and hold as you gently gaze forward.

2. Easy pose with twist (parivrtta sukhasana):

From easy pose, slide your right hand on the floor behind you, then place your left hand on the outer corner of your right knee as you twist to the right, looking over your right shoulder. When twisting, it is imperative to align your body and ensure you are lengthening your spine before going into your twist. Then do the same twist on the left side. This pose helps release stress from the body.

3. Butterfly (baddha konasana):

From easy pose, lengthen your spine as you bend your knees and bring the soles of your feet together toward your pelvis. Be mindful not to slouch as you keep lifting your chest upward. Gently hold onto your ankles, as you keep lifting your sternum up. For a deeper stretch, softly bounce your knees up and down from the floor.

4. Half-Bridge (sethubandhasana):

From butterfly, release your ankles, bend your knees and lie on your back. With your feet hip-width apart, bring your feet closer to your hips with your arms by your side. Lift your hips up as high as you can, but keep your shoulders and head relaxed on the mat while your feet and legs are parallel to each other, with heels anchored to the floor. For a deeper version, interlace your fingers beneath your lower back as you bring your shoulder blades closer together. Or, for a restorative pose, use a prop (such as a block or folded blanket) under your sacrum and allow your hips to rest on that prop. If using the block, try placing it at various heights and see which one feels the best. Benefits include a good release for the spine and chest.

5. Legs-up-the-wall pose (viparita karani):

From bridge pose, sit up and readjust your mat by placing the shorter end against the wall. Before sitting down, ensure that you have all the props you might need nearby—a bolster, blankets, eye pillow, etc. Then, sit with your left side against the wall and swing your legs up on the wall. As you lower your upper body down on your mat, wiggle your hips closer to the wall if needed, using your hands for stability. Place your arms in a T shape at shoulder level with palms facing the sky. Close your eyes as you release your legs and feel your lower body relax. This pose soothes the mind and relieves backache, tired legs and the nervous system. After about 30 seconds, bend your knees and press the heels of your feet into the wall. Then push away and roll over onto your right side of your body and lift up into a seated kneeling position.

6. Child's pose (balāsana):

From your kneeling position with hands resting on your knees, inhale and gently lean forward until your forehead touches the floor (or a block if needed). Slide your hands back, with your arms by your side and palms facing up. Tuck your chin and relax your shoulders and neck. This is an excellent pose to release tension as it also helps stretch the muscles of the lower back while it relieves the muscles of the front body.

7. Corpse pose (savasana):

This final pose is a yogi's favourite because it allows your body to transition into complete relaxation. From child's pose, simply lift back up into seated position and then lie down on your back with your feet slightly apart and arms by your side, palms facing up. Close your eyes and reconnect to your breath as you transition into deep relaxation. Hold for 1 - 2 minutes, or longer if needed.

Log on to TiffanieCarr.com for more sequences.

Yoga Breathing

Breathing is life, gives life; we wouldn't survive long without it. As mentioned by Ripa Ajmera on livestrong.com, "the ancient yogis taught that if you can learn to regulate the way you breathe, you can gain greater control over your mind as well."

You can also improve your lung capacity and your oxygen intake when you are aware of all the phases linked with breathing: the inhale, exhale and pauses between breaths. Unfortunately, only one-third of our population uses their full breathing capacity (Sivananda Yoga Vedanta Centre, 101 Essential Yoga Tips). When you don't breathe properly, it affects your whole being and can even make you feel lethargic and stressed.

Pranayama, which means "yoga breath" in Sanskrit, derives from the words "prana," meaning energy or life force and "ayama," meaning to stretch and expend. When both words are linked, they form the idea of extended breath (doyouyoga.com).

Proper breathing also keeps you present and provides the energy to move with greater ease into your practice. When your breathing is still and calm, your mind will be the same. That's one of the reasons why practicing deep and controlled yoga breathing is so beneficial.

Explore the following powerful yoga breathing techniques that will reset your mind, body and soul:

1. Sukha pranayama (also known as easy breath):

This breathing technique offers deep tranquility for the body and mind and is easy to practice anywhere, especially during stressful moments.

In a comfortable seated position, close your eyes and relax your body. Connect with your natural breath and lengthen your spine. Breathe naturally in and out through your nose and place both your hands on your belly. Be mindful of the breath travelling down to the belly and notice if your stomach expands with each inhale and contracts with each exhale. If it doesn't, this means you've been breathing from the chest, which is considered shallow breathing and isn't as powerful. Keep a peaceful mind and only notice your breathing. When inhaling, observe the energy flow inward and when exhaling, feel the stagnant energy, tension and stress leaving your body.

2.   Nadi shodhana (alternate nostril breathing):

Nostril breathing is one of the most decongesting breathing exercises in yoga. Not only does it open your nasal passages, it also reduces anxiety and helps increase mental focus, appeases the nervous system and can improve your sleep. Nostril breathing is also a perfect exercise for mind focus since it uses both the left and right nostril at the same time. I recommend practicing this technique in front of a mirror first so you get used to the hand movement in relation to the breath.

Let's begin: sitting in easy pose, place your right hand into the Vishnu Mudra hand position by bending your right middle and pointer fingers into the palm of your right hand while your thumb, ring and pinkie fingers extend. (If this is difficult, then place your hand into a water-gun pose and use your pointer finger and thumb to complete this exercise).

Start by placing your right thumb over your right nostril and take a deep inhale through the left nostril. Then, take your ring finger and bring it on top your left nostril and exhale through the right nostril. You have now completed one round of nadi shodhan pranayama.

Leave your hand as it is and immediately inhale through the right nostril. Then place your thumb over the right nostril and exhale through the left nostril. Keep the breath natural and repeat this movement back and forth without force or any pauses for a total of 9 rounds.

Tip: Each time you inhale through one nostril, switch sides to exhale in the other nostril, then inhale again and switch; repeat on the other side. Continue taking long, deep, smooth breaths without force or effort. You have the option to keep your eyes closed throughout this exercise. Make sure you have tissues nearby, as you may need them to blow your nose!

If you want to learn more about this breathing technique, log on to my website at TiffanieCarr.com.

3. Kapalabhati (breath of fire):

This breathing exercise is my favourite. It uses rapid, pumping breaths through the nose to stimulate the nervous system, purify the cardiorespiratory system (through the removal of gaseous waste) and energize the mind. You also get a nice glow after repeating this breathing exercise a few times.

Before starting, take 5 deep Sukha pranayama breaths. Next, place your hands on your belly and take one long inhale, puff up your belly and then take between 10 to 25 quick "pumping" breaths. The pumps remove the air out of your lungs by quickly contracting the muscles of your stomach. The only thing moving is your stomach. Start with practicing this breathing for three rounds and slowly increase the duration and rounds. To see the breathing exercise in action, log on to TiffanieCarr.com.

Relaxation and Meditation

For many of us, taking care of ourselves has become a low-priority task. We complain we just don't have the time as we run from one place to another looking after everyone, but ourselves. Consider this: before take-off, the pre-flight safety briefing advises travellers to put their oxygen mask on first before helping anyone else. This is an important reminder, because if you run out of oxygen, you can't help anyone. In other words, if you don't take care of yourself, nobody else will. It's time to take a moment out from your hectic schedule and recharge.

To assist you, I've compiled three powerful meditations for your much-needed peace of mind, but first a word on meditation: To get the most out of it, turn your attention inward and increase your awareness. It is important to relax and still the mind. This means sitting in a quiet space, away from distractions, is essential so you can slowly drift away from your physical space where time doesn't exist. Although you may not find blissful escape the first time you meditate, with a little patience, it will come.

A few pointers: you can sit in easy pose (cross-legged position) or use a block or bolster under your sit bones to lift your hips above your knees and ease any lower back pain. Meditating in a chair is also a popular option. Before starting any session, guide your mind to calmness and forget the past and future.

Relax your breath and use the easy-breath technique learned in the pranayama section. Let your mind roam at first, but, slowly and patiently, have an intention of focusing your thoughts on one point. Centre all your energy and attention on that. This focal point can be anything you wish: the rhythm of your breath, a mantra (a word or phrase you repeat, like "OM"), an image, etc.

Above all, make sure the thoughts that are present are supportive and positive, as every thought creates your reality. Choose thoughts that bring you joy; thank the others that don't and let those go.

Tip: Meditate for short periods of time—five minutes is a good place to begin—and gradually increase the amount of time. Let's begin:

1. Release Tension Meditation

Spine erect, begin in a comfortable seated position of your choosing. As you become still, bring awareness to your body and slow down your breathing. Choose a mantra that will benefit your current state of being. One of my favourites is "So Hum," meaning "I am that" in Sanskrit, with "that" symbolizing the universe / creation. Therefore, by repeating "So Hum", you are affirming: "I am one with the Universe and all of creation", courtesy Melissa Eisler, mindfulminutes.com.

As you count to 6 for both your inhales and exhales, slowly say your mantra as you breathe out. Notice if you have any tension in your body as you scan it from top to bottom. If you do come across any, send your breath to that area and imagine it's filled with soothing light energy. Set an intention of letting go of any other tightness and visualize all tension leaving your body. Repeat this practice until your body feels completely at ease and relaxed.

Here are four mantras (also known as prayers) that you can use in your meditation practice. Feel their uplifting energy in your body as you repeat them either out loud or in your mind:

- SA TA NA MA: This means "infinity, life, death, rebirth."
- OM NAMA SIVAYA: Some believe this mantra can help destroy ignorance as it asks God for help in transforming our destructive qualities - courtesy Atkins, 30-Day Revitalization Plan.
- OM SHANTI: This combines OM, meaning "divine energy," with the Sanskrit word Shanti, which means "peace."
- OM MANI PADME HUM: This mantra should be recited slowly because it's at the core of many Buddhists traditions. Meaning "the

jewel is in the lotus," the mantra reminds us that the lotus flower is within us all - courtesy Aimee Hughes, yogapedia.com.

2. Light Energy Meditation

Sitting comfortably, eyes closed, bring awareness to your breathing. As you come into a deeper state of relaxation, visualize yourself flying upward in the sky, like a bird, as bright white light surrounds you. Feel the positive warmth from that light radiate all its sparkling colours on you. The energy this light projects is soothing and beautiful. You instantly feel release in your entire body. Acknowledge the light's powerful presence and know deep inside this light is a reminder you are never alone and things will always work out for you. Gently start noticing your breath again and after a few minutes see yourself flying back down to earth and slowly come back to where you are at this moment. Open your eyes and breathe deeply for 5 breaths.

Last Words

As a child, I was depressed and often thought I hated life. Thankfully, I am in a much better place now, thriving as a wellness coach and yogi. I feel realigned with my purpose and I'm happy to say I LOVE LIFE! Along with yoga, I'm also a master Reiki healer and a mindfulness workshop leader. I help my clients get unstuck from the clutter in their minds, so they can achieve their health and fitness goals through a sound mind-body-soul approach. It's time to put the oxygen mask on you first. Connect with me today to learn more about my services and how I can help you feel incredible from the inside out. Visit TiffanieCarr.com to book a complimentary 20-minute phone call.

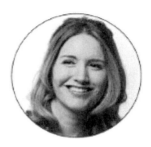

About
Ms. Tiffanie Carr

Ms. Tiffanie Carr is an energetic and passionate yoga instructor with over 2,000 hours of teaching experience. Over the years Tiffanie has taught kickboxing, boot-camp and aqua-fitness classes. Tiffanie's first love will always be Yoga, which she's been teaching since 2007. In 2017, she deepened her study of yoga under the teachings of Ron Reid and Marla Meenakshi Joy at the reputable Downward Dog Yoga Centre in Toronto. Her mission is to help people feel reconnected to their inner power through a Zen mind-body-soul approach.

Born a public speaker, Tiffanie also loves teaching workshops that empower women. Creator of Yoga on Wheels, Tiffanie travels around Toronto, giving talks to women about the importance of being mindful through meditation and yoga. As a Reiki Master, Tiffanie has been called: "A powerful Healer and a Light Worker" by her peers and clients. To learn more about her services or to book a free 20-minute call, visit TiffanieCarr.com

Chapter 15

Keeping Your Qigong Strong

By: Prof. Dr. Stanley Ngui

Qigong is a combination of two words.
"Qi" is energy and "gong" is discipline.
Together they refer to a way of life.

Let's Look at Qi

This whole universe exists because of Qi. What is energy? Energy is anything that exists, whether it is physical or non-physical.

Take the air around you, for example. You cannot see it, making it non-physical, non-visual, but you can feel it physically. Like Qi, air is both. There is a lot of energy you cannot feel, or that your senses are not aware of, but it does exist.

In respect to the whole universe, the energy we are aware of is less than a dot. That means our visual spectrum, or our sensory spectrum, is less than a dot in this whole universe of the Qi that exists in the universe.

Energy exists to sustain the universe. That's what it is; that's why the universe exists. Anything we talk about has to do with energy, whether it's vibrational energy or static energy. In Western science, there are two distinctive orders of energy.

The first energy is static. Static energy is potential energy. Then there is dynamic energy, which is kinetic energy. Almost every child is taught this in school.

Every time we do work, that's energy. That includes speaking — we have to vibrate our vocal chords to produce energy to communicate with each other. So, every single thing in this universe is energy.

Now Gong

It's translated as "discipline" and "practice." It suggests a lifestyle, something you do or are all the time. So, when you combine the words, you get energy practices.

How Do You Benefit from Qigong?

Since we are made of energy, it is important to keep it in balance. When your systems are imbalanced, it creates disorder in your body. If your body is made of energy, then you should be using energy to bring it back to where it should be.

Using energy to correct yourself; is what Qigong is all about. It is bringing good Qi back into your body and having it correct your body and bring it back to the norm, or homeostasis (balance).

The Importance of Learning

Like everything else in this world, there are aspects of Qigong that are easy to learn and can be implemented easily into your life. Other aspects can only be taught by a master.

Because Qigong involves all aspects of your life — physical, mental and spiritual — it is not something you play around with. It is something you adopt as a lifestyle. It becomes a part of you. That is why it can be very complex, because you are. It is important you have someone who is well trained in the art of Qigong to help you to determine what is the best course of action for you.

I strongly suggest you study Qigong before trying it. You also want to have a good understanding of how it works before searching out a master to work with. As with all professions, there are those who say they are masters when they are not.

What are some ways to look for a good master? Here are a few questions you can ask them.

1. How long have they been in it? A true master is someone who has done this for a long time.
2. Who were they trained under? Did they learn it by themselves or did they mentor under a master?
3. Do they have testimonies from satisfied clients? If they can't provide proof of their abilities, you do not want to go with them.

Choosing the right master and mentor is important. Misuse of Qigong can have the opposite effect to what you want. You want someone who can create a custom treatment plan for you and not do the same one for everyone.

Body-Mind Awareness

If you want to know how to use Qigong, you have to know where to start. You can't just start anywhere. First of all, you have to be aware of your body. Where are you having problems? Most people know they are sick, but they can't tell you why. It is important to be able to go beyond "I am feeling sick, I am feeling pain" to being able to accurately describe what is going on in your body. For example, instead of "My back hurts," you would say, "I am having sharp pains in my shoulder blade when I move a certain way."

Too many people wait to go to the doctor to try to figure out what is going on. That is not awareness. You can determine what and how you are feeling. It is also important to be able to pinpoint when it started.

Awareness is important in Qigong, because how will you know you are getting better if you don't know where you are starting? It is encouraging when you can notice a 50-percent improvement.

You also have to be aware of what is going on in your mind. Your mind is a powerful tool in the healing process. You must be able to control your thoughts to allow healing to come.

Most people who are chronically ill also have mental-health issues contributing to it. Depression makes it very hard to get well, because you don't believe things will ever change. For healing to come, that has to be uprooted first.

I treated a lady with cancer recently. She was very stressed, so the first thing I did, before any cancer treatment, was treat her for her mind. When she left smiling, I knew that was like 50 percent of the cancer resolution itself.

Qigong Is a Journey

Qigong, when properly used, becomes a lifestyle choice. As you use it, it becomes an unconscious part of you, but it takes time. In the beginning, it is good to set a path and goals for yourself.

One always must have a goal. The reason you have to have a focus is to know where you want to go and what you want to do; you can't be aimless all the time.

In terms of Qigong and well-being itself, the obvious goal is to be well, to be on top of the world health-wise, to be happy. Those are goals. To be free of stresses and so forth. Those are obvious goals.

How do you get there?

It is similar to sports. If you want to be the best baseball player, you determine your path, but how do you get there? You set goals and start to practice. You don't start by hitting home runs; you start by hitting the ball as far as you can and then practice, practice, practice until you are hitting it out of the park.

In Qigong, there are exercises that help you to achieve your goals. As in sports, you must practice them to become proficient at them. Each person's goals and pathways are specific to them. Everyone is on a different path and must be treated in that respect. Some may need to work on the physical more, maybe some need to work on the mental more, before they start to see results. That is why it is important to have a customized treatment plan.

Your Subconscious Mind

The subconscious mind is 95 percent of your whole mind power. The conscious mind is only 5 percent. If you stress yourself out a lot, that means your conscious mind is trying to activate the subconscious mind. Then you feel tired and everything goes down the drain.

My research has shown that the subconscious consumes twenty times more energy than the conscious mind. Once you engage your subconscious mind negatively, it's going to take you down, because you have no control of it. You really don't know it exists and it consumes so much energy it drains you completely.

You can only train the subconscious mind—you cannot tell it what to do. Take, for example, the elephant that stays where it is, even though it is tied only by a rope. When it is young, trainers keep it attached to chains that it cannot break no matter how hard it tries. As it gets older, they slowly weaken the restraint until all they are using is a rope. Because the elephant has convinced itself, it can't break through, you can now tie it with anything and it will not try to get away, even though it could do so easily.

Your subconscious is the same way. It has been trained to accept as fact things that are not true and now you are trapped in that thinking. The good news is your brain can be retrained and Qigong will help do that. You can change what is negative to positive, what holds you back to what propels you forward. It will take time.

Once you are depressed, it takes a long time to come back out of it because of your whole-body functions; your hormonal system is all fired up. Your heart is beating fast and so forth — everything is fired up.

If you are really upset, or in procrastination, or experiencing any ill effects at all, it takes a long time to recover, because your whole-body system has to come back into balance.

Try not to get yourself entangled in it, because it's hard to back out of. It takes a long time to get out of it, much longer than getting into it.

Consistency in Qigong

Qi has to flow in the body in a certain manner in order for you to be healthy. If it is disrupted at any point in time, you will be ill in whatever format it is and you won't feel good.

All of this is done automatically by your subconscious mind. You don't even know it exists. That's the hard part of it: you don't know it exists. You just know whatever you feel — you feel good or bad.

To train it, you have to do what the elephant and the elephant trainers do. Keep doing it over and over again until you can do it without thinking. That's the consistency I am looking for.

It is like martial arts. Let's say you are supposed to move your arm in a certain direction to block a punch. People who do it once or twice and think they are now a master of it, will be very sore when a punch gets past their defences and hurts them. It is the same with Qi.

I tell and show them once or twice and they think they have mastered it and then are disappointed when the results aren't there. Qi must become a part of your subconscious mind and an automatic reaction to what is happening in life. You must be consistent if you want to see results.

Procrastination

Here is something I see often. People know they need to make changes, but don't. Even though it is beneficial for them, they come up with every excuse in the book as to why they can't take action now.

I want to encourage you to not wait until it is too late. We all have a finite number of days on this earth. I have seen so many who could have led better lives if only they had not put it off.

I would love to help you. Please contact me at www.nguistyle.com and book a time to talk to me or one of my highly trained staff. I have studied under the masters in China and would love to share with you how Qi can change your life.

Don't wait until your life is miserable and you are very sick. Contact me now and we can create a custom program for you that will keep your Qi in balance.

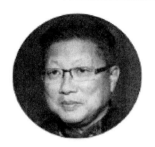

About
Prof. Dr. Stanley Ngui

Prof. Dr. Stanley Ngui is the founder of NGUI-MATRIX ™, which is a clinical technique used to treat pain and other illnesses via the brain with one touch. He is the professor at large at the World Organization of Natural Medicine ™. Part of his day is spent in treatment at the NGUI style Integrative Medicine Clinic. Some of his accolades are PhD in traditional Chinese Medicine, Doctor of Integrative Medicine, Qi Gong grandmaster, member of North America Martial Arts of Fame and knight of the Sovereign Orthodox Order of the Knights Hospitaller of St John.
www.nguistyle.com

Chapter 16

Never Give Up On You!

By: Dr. Sany Seifi

I don't remember much about this, since I was only seven months old, but my family had told me when I was a baby, I got so sick that I was on life support. Doctors couldn't do anything for me and decided to take me off all machines and let me die. When my dad got to the hospital, however, he argued with them and wouldn't let them unplug me. He then stayed at the hospital and kept praying beside me. A day passed, then I opened my eyes and started laughing loud with delight. My grandmother told me this.

The rest of my infancy proceeded smoothly. I went to school one year earlier than I was supposed to and fell in love with learning new things.

Even though we lived in a luxurious house and even had maids, I did not stop pushing myself, I continued learning new skills. Whether it was sports, books, or languages, life was great. In karate I got first place and was training for the national competition. I had two weeks to go to my big fight, then suddenly everything became dark and I could hear myself screaming, "My leg! My leg!"

When I opened my eyes five days later, I found myself in a hospital bed, vomiting. I did not recognize anyone around me; I did not understand what was going on. I couldn't move my left leg. My face was bruised and the white of my eyes was totally red.

They told me I had survived a bad car accident, but everything was okay and I went back to sleep. Two or three weeks later, I started feeling a bit better and came back to my senses. I asked, "Where are my parents and my sister?" "Your sister is beside you in the next bed." I looked at her I couldn't recognize her; her teeth were broken and she just survived a ruptured spleen.

"Your parents are in the adult section. Don't worry!" I went back to sleep. As the days passed, I became more alert and asked the nurse to bring me to my parents. The nurse now told me they had been sent to another city because they weren't in good condition. I got a bit worried and asked if they were for sure okay. And the nurse told me, "Yes, don't worry. Just pray; they will be okay."

I was really worried and kept praying and praying. One month had passed, before I could finally go home. It wasn't easy to move me around; I needed at least two people to carry me because my leg was in full plate. My femur, tibia, fibula and patella had all been fractured.

215

I was so happy to be going home and I prayed that my parents would come home soon, too. Then another month passed. I said to my aunt, "I want you guys to call the doctor, so I can talk to him about my parents' condition." They kept saying tomorrow and tomorrow, until my dad's friend came to visit a few days later and told me the truth. I would never see my parents again. They are in heaven and I should just pray for them.

All this time I had been told lies. They had lost their lives together during the car accident. I asked him, "What do you mean?" I started crying, but for less than a minute. My tears dried out, my mind went blank, my mouth got dry, my heart got cold. I noticed my left knee was stiff.

Yes, I was only eleven years old and I couldn't walk anymore, I couldn't bend my knee anymore and I was living in silence with a pain that was scarring my heart every single day. Two hours of physiotherapy daily because my knee had lost its range of motion. I had to bear the pain if I wanted to give my leg a chance and maybe get it back to normal. After a year, it was better, although I still had a limp.

It was painful to come home every day and see dad's relatives around me arguing over my dad's money and property. School was not a good place for me anymore. I decided to drop out and forget about all the money and property my dad had left behind. I would become just like him: start from the bottom and make my way up.

People around me didn't understand my pain. I was going through a big black hole, so I decided to leave the country. A few of my cousins were studying in the Philippines. I joined them and started attending school again. After a year or so I found my way through and was able to start working with the Philippines National Police. I also got into exporting Dole bananas, which was my foundation to start making my own money.

I finished one year of high school and went straight to University. I decided to live on my own because I wasn't comfortable living with my cousins.

The grief was still with me, so I started taking painkillers and sleeping pills. I didn't know the side effects of those pills; a few times I found myself in the hospital, doctors had just saved me from dying. I was drinking alcohol often and smoking cigarettes. I was lost. I couldn't find my way. I was getting old in my teenage years and gaining weight.

216

One day my cousin called to wish me happy birthday; I didn't even know it was my birthday. That was a wake-up call, for sure. I was also surprised when she said, "Oh, you are eighteen now." I had totally forgotten how old I was. I never paid attention to myself. I felt like I was forty-five.

I looked in the mirror and asked myself... What I was doing? Why am I becoming this person? I have been crying and angry and self-destructive for years now. Would that bring my parents back? No.

I realized I had been making choices I was not aware of and developed bad habits based on my choices. Do I want to look fat? Do I want to look old? Do I want people to look at me like I have no hope in life?

I was sick and tired of it. The next day I signed up at the gym. I started running, working out, trying different things, different detox pills, etc., but it wasn't working. My leg was still hurting so much; it was just rough.

One day I got constipated which lasted for two weeks. I felt like, I was dying again. I couldn't take the pain, no one was there to help me. I took a bottle of alcohol out of frustration and drank some; it started burning my stomach even more. I felt like I wanted to stab my stomach. I called my sister back home and she told me to go see a doctor.

My doctor told me I had Helicobacter pylori (H. pylori) and I must treat it with antibiotics. I had a visa for Canada, so I went and saw a doctor there who also told me I should take antibiotics as well.

I started taking them. They helped a bit, but after a few weeks everything went back to the same situation. I was getting frustrated. Everyone was telling me I looked so puffy. Nothing was helping me.

I went back to my family doctor and she sent me to a specialist. She gave me stronger antibiotics and told me I should take them for two weeks twice a day.

"So, doctor, can you please tell me why this is happening to me?" "I don't know. Some people have H. pylori and that's just how it is." "What can I do help it? Go on a special diet or anything like that?" "I don't know. You can eat anything."

I was very disappointed by this; however, I took my antibiotics for two weeks. I was getting weaker and weaker. They were really strong for my body and I had no idea how to minimize their side effects. After I finished the antibiotics, something told me to pay attention to my diet and my body, because I still wasn't feeling any better.

I became very strict with my diet and stopped eating red meat, rice, starch, sugar and anything that possibly could be a trigger. After a month of working on my diet I started feeling better and better. I noticed I was losing weight and feeling lighter and happier, so I decided to get more into it. I added fresh fruit and vegetables and ate more seafood. Then I also stopped drinking alcohol and smoking for good.

My digestion started getting better, everything was getting better. I had gone back and finished my pharmacy program in the Philippines then returned to Canada. Now I was nineteen, still kind of lost, because I realized pharmacy was not for me and I felt like it can't help people the way I wanted to. I was suffering from chronic yeast infections, which was a side effect of taking lots of antibiotics. I kept seeing different doctors and they couldn't treat it. I decided to take my own route again, which was to focus on diet and everything natural.

I started helping myself by taking more natural remedies and my yeast infection was TREATED, thank God. One day as we were driving, my brother-in-law said, "Hey, Sany. Since you are getting into a natural medicine, you might like this naturopathic medicine school. They teach medical stuff like medical schools do, but natural treatment based."

I got so excited and a few days later I visited the school. I knew this was for me. I wanted to heal, grow and help myself and others eventually. Today I'm still grateful to my brother-in-law for his suggestion.

It took me a year to get into naturopathic medicine school and say goodbye to pharmacy. It wasn't easy. I did not have a day off; the program was tough. Life was getting harder, yet sweeter at the same time. I realized I could have had a miserable life, but natural medicine saved me. It feels so amazing to be healthy and have a happy gut. I also started shadowing some naturopathic doctors and I saw first-hand how other people were getting treated with natural medicine while western medicine could not help them.

I finished my second degree at naturopathic medicine school in 2018 and I want to share some really valuable experiences and health tips,

218

especially with young people, whom I would love to inspire and help to take a natural route to staying happy, youthful and healthy.

Why Love Yourself?

Unfortunately, we are living in a world where there is not much awareness about loving and appreciating who you are. That's why we grow up not knowing how to love ourselves or be confident in our own skin and happy with our looks.

There was a long period as a teenager where I forgot about myself. I did not understand what self-love meant and how important it was for my well-being. Because of the car accident, I limped for a few years and my left leg and body were full of scars. Every time I looked at my scars it hurt. My sister suggested to laser my scars away. But I had another surgery coming up, so I had to put it off and it never happened.

I'm glad I never removed my scars. Whenever I wore a dress or shorts, people would approach me and comment on the big scar on my leg. "Omg, is that a natural tattoo?" "Were you born with this? It's so unique."

This made me rethink my scars. I realized that, indeed, they are unique. I don't see anybody else with these scars. And when you look at them, they tell you a deep story.

I started loving them so much I felt connected to them. I realized any imperfection is a sign of strength and comes with a story that is unique and often incredible, so I must love myself the way I am and embrace the natural look and the scar life has given me. My confidence was boosted. Now people make beautiful comments about my scars.

So, what really is self-love? I define it as being aware of your physical body and your soul. Once you are aware of both, you must remember your body is your own castle that nobody else has access to and your mind and soul is the type of soldiers and furniture you put in the castle. You design your own castle. So, it is very important, we are trained at an early age to be aware of that and practice building a beautiful and secure self.

I would love to see self-love as a subject in our educational system. We need to learn how to love ourselves. We grow up believing it is okay to eat all types of junk food, such as fast food and sugary stuff. Plus letting negative energy grow around our body and mind. Suddenly you are a twenty-year-old, maybe overweight, inactive, with acne, all of which causes damage to your soul and leads to anxiety, self-doubt and so on. This is where I have seen many teens developing insecurities and looking for ways to cover up their looks. They want to fix it all in one day, which isn't possible and causes further frustration.

It is my suggestion you train from an early age to love your body and love your soul. Once you eat healthy food you will end up with a healthy gut. Your gut is connected to your mind. A healthy gut equals a healthy mind and therefore you feel good in your body and have a peaceful mind.

However, let's focus more on the soul and mind. Unfortunately, modern life offers things that can play tricks on your mind and cause issues for your soul. For example, cosmetic surgery and make-up is a big attraction now. Cosmetic surgery was first used for physical deformities caused by automobile and industrial accidents. Gradually surgeons evolved their methods and now cosmetic surgery is one of the best-paid careers. Most young people want to change their looks because of their insecurities and lack of self-love, or because their peers are doing it, so they think they must do it too.

There will always be trends that you will be persuaded to go for, because you are a potential money-maker for those industries. But if you love yourself just the way you are, you will be comfortable in your own body and skin and will not let anybody use you this way.

I am sure someone has asked you, "Are you okay?" Without you telling them anything. Your energy and your waves are constantly in contact with other people around you, without you knowing it. Loving yourself works the same way. Once you love yourself and are happy with who you are, people receive that energy, that wave and are attracted to you instantly. Because self love is powerful.

Think about it. Kylie Jenner, a celebrity, started using lip fillers and brought out her own lipstick brand which made her millions, but she recently went back to her natural lips and promoting self-love and a natural look. Why did that happen when it did? Because she had grown up and learned to love her real self.

Once you love yourself, nobody can take that away from you. Your love and your energy will attract good people and good energy and you will live in peace, in a happy body and mind. If you don't love yourself, no matter what you do, you will not have pure love. If someone loves you for your big lips or your big butt, there is always a bigger butt out there. If someone loves you when you have make-up on, once the make-up is washed off, the love is washed away too. It works the same for guys as well, if a girl likes you for your big muscles what happens if you lose weight?

The question you should ask yourself is, do I want to live with my original and unique self or do I want to hide it? I hope you pick your natural self, because it is unique, it is beautiful. There is only one of you in the whole world. In the future, your baby will need your love and will look up to you to learn how to love herself. So, don't fall for industry, business and money-maker games.

Eat healthy from an early age, treat your body right and love yourself the way you are. Once you or someone else loves you for who you are, that love will never die.

Love your uniqueness. Every single part of you is unique. Brag about it and be proud of it. Don't ever let anyone tell you another version is better. Proudly love your imperfections.

Why is it Necessary to Eat Healthy from Early Age?
How Does it Affect Your Brain Health?

So many people tell themselves they will start eating healthy when they pass thirty, or forty, or when they feel ready. I'll tell you why it is not going to work as you thought it would. Just like when you plant a seed and it takes years for it to grow and become a nice tree, similarly, that is how your body works.

As you grow up, the food you put in your body will show its results later—maybe a few years later, or maybe a decade (except for food allergies, of course, whose effects are immediately apparent).

As you age, your digestion and metabolism slow down. Your energy will also decrease and there will be a change in your hormones as well. If you wait for decades to start eating healthy and then expect to see quick results—well, I wouldn't say it could never happen, but it can be frustrating and the process can be slow. It's better to start eating healthy at a young age and prepare your body for the next thirty to fifty years, so when things start to decline, it doesn't happen very fast, because your body is healthy and strong.

Your intestines are involved in a variety of bodily functions such as detoxification, inflammation management, nutrition absorption, appetite, digestion and utilization of carbohydrates and fat and energy production. What you might not know is your intestines or gut health also affects your mood, hormones, libido—even your perception of the world and the clarity of your thoughts. Nearly everything about our health and how we feel emotionally and physically can depend on the state of our gut health.

I have seen dramatic changes in mental health, skin conditions and autoimmune conditions with simple dietary changes and natural remedies that boost and support them. So, start paying more attention to your diet and what you eat.

Here Are a Few Tips on How to Have a Better and Healthier Diet for a Better Gut

1. Eat food rich in probiotics. Probiotics are good bacteria in your gut. The mechanism of their action includes the inhibition of pathogen growth, secretion of antimicrobial substances and toxin inactivation.
2. Eat fewer carbs and more fruit and vegetables. Diets high in sugar and low in fibre feed unwanted bacteria, increase the chances of intestinal permeability, cell damage and a compromised immune system and increase inflammation.
3. Drink filtered water daily. I recommend one litre as the minimum if you are not active. Drinking lots of water is important for the intestinal health, but it is also very important to drink water that does not contain chemicals and toxins, which can damage intestinal health. I recommend using household water filters, which are simple to use and inexpensive.

Why is it Necessary to Stay Active All Your Life?

You might say, "Oh, I'm not active, but I don't have this problem."

I was lucky to learn my lesson at a very young age. Inactivity started bothering me so much after the accident because my body was already used to being active. Once I became inactive, my body became unhappy and started showing symptoms. Most people are regularly inactive until their mid-thirties and since the body takes months or years to respond to good or bad habits, that's why it might not bother some people until later in life.

The point is: being active is crucial for your body and mind and must be treated as a part-time job. This way you won't let your busy life prevent you from being active. So many of my patients have told me they stopped being active in high school because they got busy with life. Now they must see a doctor every week or pay so much money for different treatments and remedies to help their condition, due to inactivity.

Being active helps your body function properly, circulating blood and bringing nutrition and oxygen to your cells to make everything in your body function better. It also helps your mood. Being active for an hour three or four times a week has been shown to work as an antidepressant. In a world full of stress and worries, is it better to be on a natural antidepressant without negative side effects? Or would you prefer to take antidepressants and be subject to weight gain, insomnia, anxiety, etc.?

That is why I think you must treat your body like it's a fancy car. Change your oil every few months (detox), turn your car on every day to protect the battery from erosion (exercise), bring your car to the car wash on the weekends to clean your car inside out (shaking off the negativity around you), drive at the speed limit (not too fast, to ward off exhaustion and not too slow, to reach your health goals before it's too late).

If you don't take care of your car, what happens? You need to spend lots of money to repair it. In a worst-case scenario, you'll need to buy a new car, but can you buy a new body? We all know the answer is no. So, treat your body right, get outside and exercise. This way you are practicing prevention and will live a good life in a strong and healthy body and mind.

I hope this chapter encourages you to rethink and start paying more attention to your body and mind. My goal was to trigger your mind and turn the key. Once you are moving, there are lots of good naturopathic doctors and great books, including my upcoming book, which will be more on health and diet tips and what to eat, to help you stay on track and reach your goals.

I would like to thank the Canadian College of Naturopathic Medicine for giving me the opportunity to heal, grow and be able to help others to heal. Also, my deepest thanks and love to my two sisters who have been to hell and back with me and were always there for me.

My 10 tips that I think helped me a lot in life and I hope they help you as well.

1. Stay true to yourself.
2. Put your health before anything else.
3. Love yourself because nobody else can love you like you do.
4. Take time to relax your body and mind and celebrate every small accomplishment in life.
5. You are the best and strongest; don't let anyone tell you any different.
6. Stay away from negativities.
7. Start your day with a smiley face and hug the people around you daily.
8. Never judge anyone, it's toxic for your brain.
9. Smile at life, regardless of what is happening to you.
10. Never forget to pray and appreciate the blessings around you, no matter how small or big they are.

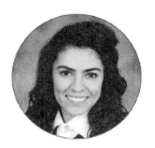

About
Dr. Sany Seifi

Dr. Sany Seifi has 3 major degrees in pharmacy, naturopathic medicine and doctor of natural medicine. She also has her PhD in natural and integrative medicine.

She is in her mid 20s and loves to make people smile and spread love with positive energy. She is very passionate about fitness and workouts everyday at least for 2 hours. She loves to travel and enjoy seeing different parts of amazing nature.

Find Dr. Sany on Instagram at @drsanyseifi or contact her at Sanyseifi@gmail.com

Chapter 17

Things Don't Happen –
People Make Things Happen!

By: Mr. Raymond Young
& Ms. Hailee Young

As you are reading through this collaborative effort, I wanted to open our chapter—and I say "our," as I have the wonderful opportunity to share this chapter with one of my four daughters—with the statement in the chapter heading. Hailee and I want to come from two perspectives, my perspective being thirty years in business, as a trainer and a coach, Hailee's as a young millennial who already, at twenty-one, has been infinitely successful in her business and leadership journey.

So, back to the opening statement. "Things don't happen—people make things happen." This idea was instilled in me from when I was a very young boy. My dad, with all his faults—we all have them—was amazing at teaching his children how to survive. The thing I am most thankful for is how he simplified everything.

As a young boy, I watched him intently. He was my hero when I was growing up. So, when he made statements like the one above, I always listened to understand rather than listened to hear. The first thing I would like to share with you today as you are reading: listen to understand. As the words come to life on these pages, find the meaning and apply it to your day-to-day life.

Hailee and I are hopeful that we can give you some simple tools and tips to make this easier. In my thirty-plus years in business I, just like most of us, found that my habits got the most of me. You know the ones: where you intend to sit on the couch for just five minutes and five minutes turns into fifty and so on . . . or you end up involved in a conversation that is negative and doesn't serve you or the other person in the discussion.

This, unfortunately, can be covered by one simple word . . . LIFE! I'm sure you have heard it, but I will say it again here. No matter what you do, no matter how good you are and how great things can be, life keeps moving on.

To share with you a few simple tips that fundamentally changed my life and my family's legacy, to make this point clear and accurate, I need to share a couple of things. Due to my dad's teachings, from which came my infinite understanding of the word "commitment," and my work ethic, I was highly successful at a very young age. By the time I was twenty-five, I was a millionaire. By age twenty-eight, I was filing for bankruptcy and going through a divorce. This is important, because it's in the moments of tragedy that we learn to either define ourselves or lose ourselves. All too often, there's no coming back if we get lost.

So, there I was, twenty-eight years old, thinking I owned the world and then I had to start a new career and move in with my mom with my three daughters. I was in that place called "lost." The only thing I was certain of, was I did not want to stay there!

In spite of how much will I had and how much I wanted to fix my life, my habits and my fears were stopping me. The first thing I did was start to surround myself with people who were positive and outgoing. Although I would love to tell you that is the secret, that wasn't the secret.

All these people talked about reading books, listening to audio programs, self-development and so many other things. I was never a reader and I didn't want to be one of those people who went to motivational and self-help seminars. But then it happened. I heard a guy at one of those seminars that I was never going to go to say that although he hated reading, he figured he could read a chapter a day. When he said it, my immediate thought was, "You're a better man than me."

But I could read one page a day. The first new habit, the first step to changing my life, was the decision I made inside my head in a room with 10,000 people.

Here's what you need to know: I made a contract with myself. Right there in that moment, I made an agreement with myself that for five years I would read one single page, each and every day, of something positive and inspirational. I said that even if I was sick, tired, sad, frustrated, or angry, the one page was going to happen.

It's funny how life works. It was not long before I broke the agreement—I was reading multiple chapters a day. I am sharing this with you as part of our chapter because no matter what you do in life, there comes a time to commit. That commitment has to surpass anxiety, fear and any possible excuse you could make. As Muhammad Ali said, "I hated every minute of training, but I said, 'Don't quit. Suffer now and live the rest of your life as a champion.'"

Ironically enough, in and around the same time all of this was happening to me, I was watching a movie you may know, with Tom Hanks and Meg Ryan, called Sleepless in Seattle. There's a scene in the movie where the Tom Hanks character ends up on a therapist's radio talk show. He had recently lost his wife and become widowed. In the end the therapist asked Tom's character "What are you going to do now?"

Although I am paraphrasing his answer, he replied, "I'm just going to get up everyday and put my feet on the floor." This turned out to be a very profound statement for me. What I didn't know was it would become my daily mantra. Every morning when I opened my eyes, the first words I heard in my head were "I'm just going to put my feet on the floor."

Today, twenty-plus years later, there's not a single morning my eyes don't open with a positive reinforcing mantra. As Hailee takes over to complete this chapter and share some of her insights and tips, I want to clearly identify two life-defining actions.

Number 1. Fill your brain daily with something positive. One page, one video, one something powerful.

Number 2. Create a mantra. Before you allow anything distracting or upsetting to settle, open your eyes and repeat a rhythmic mantra as part of your routine.

This is where I pass the baton to my daughter Hailee.

I am thrilled to be writing this chapter with my business partner, mentor and father. In the last twenty-one years I have learned how to fall apart and how to rebuild and move forward.

Mental health has never been something that came easily to me. At a young age I was diagnosed with what seemed like every mental illness possible, from depression to anorexia to anxiety to borderline personality disorder. I began to feel like my mind was my own worst enemy, like I was in a constant battle with myself, my own consciousness being the war zone.

I was told it wasn't my fault, I had an illness. Those words were said by doctors and therapists throughout my whole childhood and although their intentions were to comfort me, it actually ended up making things worse. If it wasn't my fault, then how could I fix it?

This began a vicious cycle of living with a victim mentality, where I didn't take responsibility for anything going on in my life, good or bad. This is dangerous; how are you supposed to feel proud and fulfilled if you can't take credit for all the amazing things you have created in your life and how are you supposed to change the negative things if you believe they aren't your fault? This is where my dad's mantras and habits came in and saved me.

Something I was lucky to learn from both my parents is everything that has happened in your life has a direct link to your choices. Once I really understood this, things started to change for me. I made a commitment to start doing daily mantras and to change my negative habits into positive ones, even though that wasn't always easy.

What I learned, too, is that to make changes in your mental well-being, there has to be an improvement in your physical well-being. But even more complex a concept is that in order for you to take the initiative to make physical-health changes, your mind has to be in a healthy place.

This is where I got stumped. My original thought was that to make my emotions stable and healthy, I should make my body stable and healthy. However, when I would attempt to execute a healthy plan involving all-natural supplements, healthy eating and more water consumption, I found my mental state and bad habits would stop me from doing what I set out to do. I would take the vitamins for a week before I would give up, because taking three to five supplements three times daily was just too much in a busy life like mine. I would try to drink more water, but most times I'd forget, so I'd end up drinking litres at a time and would feel sick and spend the next hour using the washroom. This also wasn't something I could commit to long-term.

Can you relate to any of this? If so, this chapter is perfect for you.

Over time, with several failed attempts, restarts and disappointments, I have gotten down how to change your mental and physical health with little to no effort. I learned really quickly the harder your routine is, the quicker you will quit it and if you quit before it becomes a habit, then, really, it never did anything for you except teach you that it's okay to let yourself down. Your plan must be so easy that even you can't talk yourself out of it.

For me, this started with asking "How can I do what I'm already doing, but make it healthier for my mental and physical well-being?" I started to analyze my daily routine and with a little trial and error, came up with an easy-to-follow three-step plan.

#1: I switched all my products that contained harsh chemicals, from cleaners to shampoo, to all-natural ones. Our body's largest organ is the skin, so why do we believe it is okay to put chemicals on it that we wouldn't dare to ever put in our mouth?

This did not require anything extra in my daily routine, but it significantly cut the amount of toxins I came in contact with every day. These toxins have been linked to illnesses and decreased cognitive function. How is your body and mind going to work at their optimal best if they're constantly trying to fight and protect you against toxic chemicals? This was the first step to changing my physical and mental health.

#2: I got my body into an alkaline state. Right off the bat, I had been drinking a cup of coffee every morning, which instantly puts your body into an acidic state. Illnesses are grown in an acidic state, but not in an alkaline one.

I wasn't willing to give up my morning coffee, however, so I had to find ways to balance that out. That's when I discovered vitamin-infused coffee with fulvic acid by ShopPal. The fulvic acid helps balance out the acidity in the coffee and it gives me my first dose of vitamins first thing. The fulvic acid also increases my body's oxygen levels substantially, giving me even more energy than I've ever gotten from a cup of coffee. These small changes in my physical health are what gave me the energy and strength to completely change my mental health.

#3: I took vitamins, vitamins and more vitamins—my best ally and worst enemy. Because our food lacks vital nutrients, it's extremely important we take some sort of vitamin supplement. Easier said than done, right?

Because of digestion problems I developed when I was struggling with my eating disorder, most supplements give me really bad stomach pains. I was not willing to accept excruciating pain every morning, but I knew if I wanted to be healthy, I would need to find a way to get more nutrients.

I also wasn't willing to commit to the 'One pill 3x daily with meals" routine. Once I leave the house, that's it . . . there will be no more supplement-taking. However, to get the most out of your vitamins, it's important to have a steady intake through the day, as your body will expel whatever is not needed at that exact time. Ever use the washroom after you've taken vitamins and it looks like a highlighter has exploded in your toilet? That's those expensive vitamins being flushed away.

Knowing this, but not having a solution was a struggle for a long time. I spent lots of money on pills I never ended up finishing, until I found transdermal vitamin patches by PatchMD. Their slow-release formula works throughout the day, so it means one two-second application in the morning will give me more vitamin absorption than taking the equivalent pill three times a day.

I also no longer have to worry about whether it will hurt my stomach.

This became a habit really quickly for me. As my vitamin-infused coffee is brewing I take all of two seconds to apply the quarter-sized multi-vitamin patch and that's it for the day.

They completely revolutionized my health. Within six weeks of using the patches, my vitamin levels went from low to perfect. My energy also skyrocketed, along with my ability to fight off germs and illnesses. When everyone around me is getting the flu, I might get the sniffles. Being able to avoid taking time off during cold and flu season keeps my stress at bay, which helps both my physical and mental health.

These three things did not change my daily routine in any way, shape, or form. I was just taking what I was already doing and making it healthy.

Since then, my energy has improved, my stomach problems have almost completely subsided and my mental health has made huge leaps during a time I didn't think it was possible. As my physical health improved and I had more energy and mental clarity, I noticed it was easier to remember my mantras, one of my favourites being "This too shall pass." I also noticed myself actually wanting to do things that improve my mental health, like read or start a new hobby or declutter my house.

This journey is not over and I will continue to learn from others always, but without these initial steps to improve my physical health, I wouldn't have been able to improve my mental and emotional health and I certainly would not be writing a chapter in this book with so many incredible people.

If I could give any last words of advice, it would be that you need to believe you are in control of your life. Once you know you're in control, you can take small steps toward big changes.

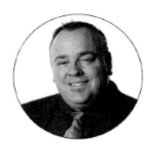

About
Mr. Raymond Young

After going through a divorce and trying financial times, **Mr. Raymond Young** went on to build one of the largest network-marketing businesses in North America. His thirty-year career has focused on training, developing and mentoring individuals. He is responsible for inspiring thousands of people through conferences, seminars and public-speaking engagements.

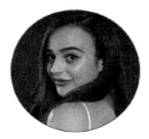

About
Ms. Hailee Young

Ms. Hailee Young is a young, female, entrepreneur who is passionate about health, wealth and animal welfare. Hailee started her career as a financial advisor at just 18-years-old and within her first year she became the youngest six figure earner in the company.

Since then, Hailee has now added two ventures, one is building a company with her father, Raymond that supports non-profits and the other being the managing director for The Bryan & Amanda Bickell Foundation. Hailee hopes that by sharing her passion for health and animals she can help make the world a better place.

Chapter 18

Feeding the Five Senses

By: Mr. Benjamin Stone

A Conscious Deep-Impact Journey toward Stepping Back into Your Full Power

As you will come to read and understand more clearly in the days, weeks and years that follow, quantum science and our evolving understanding of the universe will become part of the mainstream and you will understand and discover your hidden yet innate ability to step fully into your divine self and transform all parts of your life.

I also focus in this chapter on shifting from "dis-eased" states of being to wellness and thriving.

I want to define a few points early on, such as holism in natural medicine. It is imperative to understand that one of the fundamental differences in traditional natural medicine is we observe the body, mind and spirit of the individual. Therefore, even though it seems at times that serving only the body in its ill state yields healing results, it is truly a culmination of body, mind and spirit that is required to heal.

To benefit the most from this journey, you are advised to keep an open mind. Let's recall the history of the nineteenth-century human: burning psychics and anyone who did not conform to the ideology of the day at the stake for thoughts and capabilities of the energic realm. Society at this time were unable to fathom the insanity, at the time, of a nuclear bomb, DNA, cell phones, computers or AI, let alone the concept that everything is energy and can influence us negatively or positively.

If you expand the limits of your belief, I promise you a world limited only by your beliefs. The magic and power of understanding your role in this journey called life as more than a random individual imprisoned in the modern-day slavery of working to merely survive and begging mercy from outside sources to help you with your declining health, is yours. If I may offer you an opportunity to understand your way to self-sovereignty, take it with an open mind.

It is important to note that the allopathic medical community today is said to take an average of twenty years to bring current scientific data and understanding into the medical texts doctors graduate with. The incredible work of people like Dr. Bruce Lipton, Dr. Joe Dispenza, Dr. Amit Goswami and Joe Whalen and such early pioneers of quantum physics like Niels Bohr, Max Planck, Albert Einstein and Werner Heisenberg, to name a few and thought leaders like those above, including Alan Watts and Dr. David Hawkins, are now just seeping into the fray and finding themselves in such higher education facilities like Quantum University, training the doctors of the future.

The information contained in theses pages is part of my journey to discovery and fulfilling my purpose as a natural and integrative medicine doctor and a lecturer on energy medicine. Upon completing my PhD, I hope to have pushed the envelope a little bit further and bring up the bottom to the middle, so humanity can take back its innate power to transform their lives.

Today, many believe its mere luck or coincidence that anything good happens to us. We may even believe the gods or something outside ourselves cause the hurts and traumas we experience. Others simply believe that action, even to the degree of pushing oneself, is how we achieve anything.

I am here to say that action is the vehicle and must be employed with consistency; beliefs, mindset and emotions (resonating at an energy frequency) are the driving force that makes the difference between a long and endless struggle and a journey that happens much more effortlessly.

Deciding which fuel to put in your action vehicle is based on understanding an important quantum scientific data point that states and to quote Max Planck, "I regard consciousness as fundamental. I regard matter as a derivative from consciousness." What this means is that matter, the reality you observe as physical on this 3D plane, is constructed upon perception. In other words, reality is nothing more than an illusion, a process by which a wave form collapses unto itself to become a particle.

For 100 years quantum physics has explained that subatomic entities like electrons and photons behave as either particles (matter) or waves depending on the presence (or absence) of an observer—the human mind, consciousness, which I call the transmutation device. When one observes their behaviour using measuring instruments, they appear as particles. But when the instruments are removed, they behave like waves, meaning they do not seem to be in any specific point in space at any given moment. Unobserved, they are theorized to exist in a "superposition," the range of all locations that will be possible for them to appear in when they are observed. They do not exist in space or time, until they are observed. They literally are dependent upon the presence of the conscious mind to attain a position in three-dimensional reality.

Why is this important to understand? Because it is the ticket to your first day of realization that life does not happen to you and that you are absolutely a co-creator, at a minimum, in your reality. This offers you a basic understanding that healing and thriving—the subject of this book—depends on the subset of filters (beliefs) you observe in the quantum field (multiple and infinite) possibilities. And although the subject of life beyond the five senses is very much a topic of scientific focus for me, I want to guide you to understand how to better your life in this 3D journey, be it in relation to an illness or simply maintaining a long and thriving life.

One more way of understanding this information before we get to feeding the five senses is: everything is energy. You and everything around you is nothing more than energy. As you most likely now understand, we and everything around us, are made up of atoms. When observed under the microscope, atoms are made up of mostly invisible energy. A vast amount of empty space. Every person and object you observe has their own unique energy signature. This also goes for every single thought, belief and word.

The work of Dr. Bruce Lipton, PhD—in short, going from being an atheist one minute to believing in a higher power the next—centres on every cell of the human body being influenced by an energy, a consciousness, that goes beyond mere physicality. Antennae have been found upon each cell that are unique to the person they came from. Such observations have been found with transplant recipients receiving information and dreams about the life of the deceased donor without ever knowing them. It has also been observed cancer cells revert to healthy cells when their environment (called in biology as the medium) is changed to a healthy one.

Our beliefs filter our experience of this world and our power is that we can change them. The rub, which I believe is going to get more and more easily undone as we progress in the field of consciousness and quantum physics, is that, for the most part, our belief systems have been programmed into us from birth to age seven. During this time our consciousness has not come online and we are merely programming our subconscious (like a data warehouse tape recorder) until our conscious mind comes aboard. The subconscious that we do not have direct access to makes up 95 percent of our thoughts, with only 5 percent of the conscious mind observing. Depending on the programming you received from your parents, environment, observation, etc., you are chained to the automatic beliefs 95 percent of the time as you move through life.

The brain, through the senses, is able to take in 11 million bits (of information - the digital unit of measure for a computer of binary computations) every second, from one's environment; however, the conscious mind is only able to process a mere fifty bits (of information) per second. It is understood that the information is filtered down to match the belief systems we have. It is believed that the 100 billion brain cells are responsible for the compression of 11 million bits of information down to approximately 50 bits of information that the conscious mind can handle. Based on the conscious mind's limitations, the vast majority of processing occurs outside of one's consciousness. This means we are limited or imprisoned by our programming. Fundamentally, changing your programming through feeding the five senses with new and better nutrition has the science-backed potential to make new observations in the quantum field, bringing you a life vastly different from the one you are experiencing.

We understand that, since everything exists as a waveform before it is observed (decoded by the human brain / consciousness) and then becomes a particle (matter) we interpret as solid or physical, to change our reality we must change the resonant frequency of our emotions, our beliefs and our thoughts, along with our actions, to collapse wave forms of the infinite quantum potentialities into the particles we want to experience in our life.

There is a plethora of data on this. Below I provide an example, in simple terms to be applied to any situation, such as a current health issue. Reviewing my definition of holism at the beginning of this chapter will help you remember that no one said we are wishing away the state we are in, but through action along with changes in resonant frequency we will yield the observed quantum possibility we are seeking. Remember, acting on the physical aspects as well as the mental, emotional, spiritual is necessary to heal.

Let's say you are 250lbs and you want to be 150lbs instead. There's a 100lbs gap between where you are right now and where you would like to be. It is highly unlikely that a 100lbs weight loss is going to manifest in your body and observed on your scale today. However; you could close the gap between the feeling of being unhealthily overweight (fear, worry, anxiety) and the feeling of thriving at your ideal and healthy weight (ease, freedom, happiness) today. This, you can accomplish in five minutes. It is only a vibrational change you must make. Then those pounds must begin to shed. It is law! Many in the new thought revolution have called this the Law of Attraction. In Quantum Mechanics we would refer to this as collapsing the waveform.

You may wish to research and understand Dr. Hawkins's Map of Consciousness. Dr Hawkins suggests there are different resonant frequencies (energy) for every state of consciousness or emotion, as well as disease state. Additionally, the work of Dr Royal Rife shows pathogens also have different vibrational frequencies. With this in mind and understanding that the classic "negative" emotions and pathogens and diseased states are lower vibrations and positive emotions and states of higher consciousness and thriving health are higher vibrations, we can extrapolate this into the world of feeding the five senses that states in order to achieve optimal wellness in all areas of your life; you must take accountability and action in making informed decisions.

Feeding the Five Senses - Sight, Sound, Smell, Taste and Touch

Knowing that all matter is a frequency and resonance, we must consider the implications of feeding our five senses with the highest frequency we can; to influence our physiology into higher states of wellness and awareness. Knowledge is power, power is perception and perception offers us the quantum possibilities to uplift ourselves into a life of divine self-sovereignty.

SIGHT: The Faculty or Power of Seeing

Sight is by far the most abundant sense and accounts for up to 80 percent of our perceptions.

An example of visual perceptions that can negatively affect your physiology and well-being is blue light in the evening, which has been shown to negatively affect your circadian rhythms (for restful and restorative sleep essential to health and healing) and contribute to eye strain, cataracts, macular degeneration and even cancer.

A simple and helpful tip is to stop using blue-light technology in the evening, especially after the sun has gone down, or to use blue-light-blocking filters on your electronic devices. An inexpensive and healthful option is to buy blue-blocking glasses.

Since the 1960s, we have been compiling research and data that shows observing violence in your daily reality and according to article PMC270415 in the National Institutes of Health, as well as a report from the National Institute of Mental Health, in television shows, movies, video games, on cell phones and on the internet increases the chances you:

- May become less sensitive to the pain and suffering of others;
- May be more fearful of the world around you;
- May be more likely to behave aggressively in harmful ways toward others.
- It suggests there is a preponderance toward violent behaviour.

Violence according to Dr David Hawkins falls below the 200 line into the Levels of Falsehood.

What this does to our wellbeing and physiology is to activate our stress response, which in turn suppresses our immune system.

In response to the question of wellness and resonating to a higher vibration for our well-being, we can do simple things like walk in nature or observe the sun setting. It has been shown the effects of observing green in nature improves depressive states. Observing beautiful colours, events and acts of love and kindness causes calming chemicals to be released from the brain's pharmacy, which also activates the parasympathetic nervous system, a requirement for rejuvenation and healing.

A quote by Moira Bush (www.moirabush.com) on colour therapy:

Colour helps you to express what you cannot yet say or ready to reveal. When you feel depressed, you wear purple, when you feel powerless you wear black and when you have financial issues you wear red. Each part of your body is connected to a colour frequency that comes from the sun, certain parts of your body absorb specific colours and this is known as the chakra system. Sir Isaac Newton discovered that when he put sunlight through a prism, it created the rainbow.

When you have a period of stress or you demand a higher performance from your body, mind or emotions, you will automatically begin to crave the colour related to the body area you are focusing on and desire to add that colour through decor, food, drink or clothing. For example: when your heart is emotionally bruised, you will crave spinach and suddenly want to wear a green t-shirt, even though green is not your favourite colour. If you are in a new relationship and the sex is highly active, you will crave orange and coral colours for sexual energy, physical stamina and sensuality.

Each colour has a positive and a negative side, the positive indicates the potential and the negative indicates where the healing is needed. For example: The colour pink indicates that you are in a healthy relationship with yourself and in a romance with someone else, in the negative pink highlights unresolved mother issues and deeply buried anger and frustration from childhood. Wearing certain colours will lead to specific outcomes - wear the pink and someone will ask you out on a date! Wear pink on your next visit to your mother and watch the fall-out that releases suppressed emotions!"

HEARING: The Faculty of Perceiving Sounds

As defined by Oxford, sounds are vibrations that travel through the air or another medium and can be heard when they reach a person's or animal's ear.

Perhaps the area of most concern is what is termed noise pollution, or excessive noise. Studies have shown this can be found in environments such as offices, construction sites and even in our homes. The city's hustle and bustle in and of itself contains much noise pollution.

Its effects are evident in disturbed emotional balance, headaches, anxiety and stimulation of violent behaviour. It is also related to disturbance of sleep, constant stress and fatigue leading to lowered immunity, healing loss and cardiac issues of hypertension and increased heart rate.

It has also been noted regular exposure to loud noise decreases the ability to read and learn. Cognitive function decreases due to an inability to recall along with a decline in problem-solving capabilities. Lastly, noise pollution can lead to communication issues, which can further complicate one's relationships.

Sound therapy — exposing yourself to environments where you can decompress in silence or harmonious sounds — is key to feeding your hearing sense and raising your well-being. Nature and natural settings again rank high on the list of healthy options where the nature and its coherent sounds are healing to the body. Sounds of nature, as well as pleasant music releases neuro-chemicals that are calming, healing and regenerative and helps to improve sleep by activating the parasympathetic nervous system for rejuvenation.

SMELL: The Ability to Detect Odours or Scents

Odour or scents are detected by means of the organs in the nose, also known as the olfactory system. Considered the most primitive of the senses, smell connects us with memories, emotions and instincts. We absorb some of its molecules, making aromatherapy, for example, a form of natural medicine.

Where might we be making unevaluated and potentially damaging choices for our well-being through smell? Environmental pollutants. These pollutants are known to alter the chemosensory systems of both smell and taste senses. According to a National Institutes of health publication https://www.ncbi.nlm.nih.gov/pubmed/1608635

"Acute and chronic alterations in taste and olfaction are related to solvents, herbicides, fungicides, pesticides, disinfectants, germicides, soil fumigants, dyes, pharmaceuticals, textile wastes, smog, tobacco smoke, perfumes, flavours, plastics, synthetic rubber and other industrial substances.

Additionally, naturally occurring substances like mold and their related mycotoxins can make far-ranging and dangerous changes to your total physiology. It is not just that there can be acute, chronic, or permanent damages to the chemosensory systems; many of these substances can affect any part of your physiology, especially the brain and downregulate your body's natural abilities to detoxify (remove endogenous and exogenous toxins from the body)."

If you have been exposed to these pollutants, the very first step on the journey to healing is removing the source. It is essential to seek the advice of a knowledgeable professional in the protocols most effective for detoxification for the different substances. For example, it is important to understand mycotoxins from mold will not simply leave the body. They are notorious for downregulating a very important detoxification gene called the NRF2 protein-transcription factor.

Let's now feed the smell sense with something uplifting by first removing the substances mentioned above from your environment and

246

incorporating healthy solutions like high-quality pure essential oils. Perhaps some calming essential oils like lavender, sandalwood, neroli and vanilla.

Making delicious foods, buying and planting flowers in your garden (which, by the way, will also feed the sense of touch, smell and sight and even taste if you plant edibles) will feed your sense of smell with delight and uplifting feelings

TASTE: The Ability to Perceive Flavour in the Mouth

Oxford defines it as the sensation of flavour perceived in the mouth and throat on contact with a substance.

As mentioned under smell, there are chemicals, environmental pollutants and "accepted" food additives found in processed foods and restaurant meals that lead to many adverse health conditions. Here are just some of the big guns in the food-additive category and their health effects according to Healthline.com
https://www.healthline.com/nutrition/common-food-additives#section12

Artificial sweeteners; HFCS (high-fructose corn syrup); MSG/E621 - monosodium glutamate; trans fat; food dyes like blue #1 and #2 E133, red #3 and #40 E124, yellow #6 E110 and yellow tartrazine E102; sodium sulfite E221; sodium nitrate/sodium nitrite; BHA and BHT E320; sulfur dioxide E220; and potassium bromate.

Known Health Effects of These Additives:

Neurotoxicity, carcinogenic, decline in intelligence, brain tumours, lymphoma, diabetes, multiple sclerosis, Parkinson's, Alzheimer's, fibromyalgia, chronic fatigue, emotional disturbances such as depression and anxiety, headaches, migraines, seizures, nausea, mental confusion, high LDL (bad cholesterol), excitotoxicity, eye damage, obesity, behaviour problems, reduction in IQ, kidney and adrenal gland tumours, nerve damage, asthma, rashes, cardiac arrest, hypotension, anaphylaxis, breathing problems, thyroid dysfunction and last, but not least, nutrient depletion.

Simple Solution: REMOVE ALL THESE ADDITIVES FROM YOUR LIFE

You can boost the taste senses by incorporating all the different types of tastes found in whole foods—a mostly plant-based diet including a healthy portion of raw foods.

TOUCH: The Ability to Perceive Through Skin Contact

Touch is when external objects or forces have contact with the body, especially the hands; only sight and touch allow us to locate objects.

This is a special sense in that we require touch to maintain a healthy immune system. We need to look at the health challenges associated with not just lack of touch, but also the additives and chemicals found in environmental pollution and some soaps, gels, pastes, make-up, perfumes, body butters and creams and hair products, not to mention cleaning supplies (which also affect the olfactory system—smell). And let's not forget clothing.

The top additives that need to be avoided as much as possible:

Parabens, synthetic colours, fragrance, phthalates, triclosan, sodium lauryl sulfate, sodium laureth sulfate, formaldehyde, toluene, propylene glycol and sunscreen chemicals.

They have been shown to cause the following attacks upon our health and wellbeing by:

Estrogen mimicking; breast tumours; carcinogenicity; ADHD; allergies; dermatitis; respiratory distress; reproductive dysfunction; early breast development; birth defects; endocrine disruption; bacteria resistance; skin, lung and eye irritation; fetal damage; immune system toxicity; cellular damage; and cancer.

As you can see, there are major health issues with many of the accepted, government-approved products available for human consumption. This is where it is extremely important to fully understand your power to elevate your consciousness.

Your first order of business is to remove these additives from your life.

Additionally, feeding your touch sense with healthy touch has been shown to stimulate both serotonin and dopamine, reducing depression, anxiety and stress, lowering blood pressure and lowering cortisol levels. It has also been shown to increase bonding, lessen fidgeting, result in 82 percent less crying among hugged babies, reduce the incidence of ADHD, improve the immune system and reduce aggressive and violent behaviours.

Remember to honour your spirit with a communion of feeding your five senses with the highest vibrational foods, a healthy environment, exercise, positive relationships, silence or healthy sounds, conversations and making love. Cuddling with your loved ones, even the furry ones can provide incredible benefits. Remember, one of the most important points to remember is you must control your mind, your consciousness and your thoughts and emotions along with taking action to remove lower vibration onslaughts to your body, mind and spirit. Then, adding in the highest vibratory choices you can.

In natural medicine, some therapies to investigate to help you feed the five senses are sound therapy, light therapy, colour therapy, body work—like massage, reiki, rolfing, chiropractic, going to a raw-food retreat, or hiring a nutritionist, energy medicine including energy psychology and rife and biofeedback machines. There are many options available. Find the ones that fill your spirit and guide you to higher vibrations.

In short, the simplicity of feeding the five senses is being consciously aware of each and every choice you make. Ask yourself if your senses are being fed the best nutrition possible at any given moment.

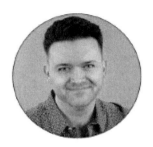

About
Mr. Benjamin Stone

My name is **Mr. Benjamin Stone**. I am an Integrative Medicine Practitioner and a Practitioner of Humanitarian Services, a Health Educator, Plant-based Nutritionist, Old Soul Empath, Intuitive Psychic Medium, Researcher, a Healer in Energy Modalities, Core Health Facilitator and currently working on my PhD in Natural Medicine based on Quantum Physics.

The basis of my work will begin with a Holistic Health Consultation comprising of an extensive in-take form and process so that I can become as deeply knowledgeable about your histology, your stresses, deficiencies, areas of wellness, diagnosed diseases, general wellness as well as your intended goals. The intention of the Holistic Health Consultation is to present your intended goals and desires and to formulate a strategy and protocol to guide you to your ultimate wellness. I can be reached at www.healtheducator.ca or by email at bstone@healtheducator.ca

Chapter 19

Breathe in Chi and Healing,

Breathe Out Negativity

By: Master Teresa Yeung

How Energetic Do You Feel Today?

Chi or Qi is the energy that is also recognized as the life force that flows through life, or the 'Tao' force. Chi encompasses the dichotomy of yin and yang; the feminine and the masculine, cold and hot. Balance is a fundamental principle of Chi, or Qi. The practice of Chi Gong harmonizes the body and the flow of energy within the body and improves your equanimity and ability to remain centred and balanced. The regular practice of Chi Gong dissipates negativity and pessimism.

Beyond discussing physical exercise to build muscle tone and flexibility, I will show you some techniques and visualizations to help harmonize and balance the mind and body. Further Chi Gong exercise and consistent practice with me will give you stronger results. Chi Gong can be used to decrease fatigue, maintain health, promote wellness, support better sleep, lower blood pressure, strengthen digestion and improve mental clarity well into old age.

Do you wish to feel more energized and balanced now? Please follow me and I will show you a few simple yet useful ways to recharge yourself easily and effortlessly.

Method One
Breathing

The fastest way to harmonize, balance and re-energize the body and mind is by learning how to move the life force, Chi* or Qi* in your body. When we're not feeling good because of negativity, stress, or disease, sitting down regularly to quietly move the energy for ten to fifteen minutes will give you good results. A Chi Gong form has more steps and deliberate movements combined with slow breaths and visualization. This is a simpler visualization technique practiced with a few breaths:

1. Breathe in with the nose and breathe out with the nose. You can visualize breathing in good energy and then breathing out negative energy. You can also visualize deliberately breathing in lots of oxygen and breathing out your fatigue and frustrations through the bottom of your feet for a couple of minutes. Visualize bright energy coming in and visualize murky or grey energy leaving your body.

If you do this, you will feel better immediately.

Method Two
Balance Psychic Centres in Your Body

Let's experiment with how to feel better by balancing different centres in your body today.

Breathing

Relax and sit quietly for a few minutes, gently closing your eyes and breathing in through the nose and breathing out through the nose. For the best energy flow, it will help if you put your tongue gently on top of the palate behind the teeth. You may not be very used to doing this at the beginning. Loosening your jaw like this bridges the chi between your mouth and your skull so it will continue to flow down the body easily. You will also create more saliva, which aids in digestion.

Choose a Practice Position

There are three practice positions for accommodation and accessibility. Most Chi Gong forms have a recommended position. For this form, you can use the one that works best for you:

1. Sit comfortably in a chair, your arms relaxed and palms facing up.
2. Lie down with your arms at your side.
3. Stand up and drop your arms to your side.

This has some visualization techniques and the pictures below are for healing in a seated position.

Three Psychic Energy Centres

Chi Gong originated in China many thousands of years ago. Many ways, forms and practices were developed to strengthen and balance the body and mind for health and longevity. By moving the Chi through visualization, combined with gentle and soft movements, as well as deliberate breathing, different Chi Gong forms with movements can support specific body parts. My Eye Chi Gong is very popular among the young and old to improve vision, sleep, headaches, focus and memory. My Overall Health & Fitness Chi Gong is simple, effortlessly loved and practiced by thousands giving you lots of good energy. You, too, can attain the benefits of Chi Gong practice.

Here is a simple way to recharge your batteries.

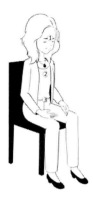

1. Head Centre

The first area is the brow area. Behind the brow is the pineal gland. The pineal gland is one of the smallest organs in the body and many consider it to be the ethereal third eye. Regardless of whether the pineal gland contributes to our intuitive functioning, it plays an important role in the body and affects our immune system. The pineal gland starts shrinking in adulthood.

2. Chest Centre

The second area is the heart, or chest centre. The heart centre is very important, as our heart never stops beating to give life. You understand the heart organ is at the centre of the circulatory system and supplies oxygen and nutrients to the tissues, working in complete harmony with the rest of the body to remove waste and carbon dioxide. Our body is a magnificent symphony of organ systems, tissue and cells. It's important we treat our bodies with love.

In ancient Egypt, it was believed the heart rather than the brain was the source of wisdom, memory and the personality itself. When someone passed away, the heart was never removed from the body during mummification and was said to be given back to the deceased in the afterlife.

The heart is the bridge to the energy of the lower and higher parts of the body. Metaphorically speaking, the heart is where we recognize our feelings of love, joy and sadness and it paints our life with beauty, compassion and love.

3.   Lower Abdominal Centre

The third area is the sacral area, or lower Dan-tien in Chinese. We will refer to this area as our core energy. It is closely connected to our reproductive energy and feelings of centeredness. Like electricity, we need a line for grounding. As we are bombarded by all the electrical devices emitting frequencies of different sorts, it's more important than ever we ground our energy.

When you are feeling balanced, you have energy, compassion, equanimity, intuition, a sense of stability and a zest for life.

How to Move the Qi or Chi

The chi goes to where your mind is. All you have to do is to start moving the Chi with deliberate breaths and visualization. You may consider gently closing your eyes to rest at the same time or practice with half-closed eyes. Healing is really just under your nose.

1.   Breathe in and visualize the universal Qi coming down, reaching your crown, flowing into your head. Breathe out and continue to let the energy flow down and out of the head centre (1). As the energy flows, visualize you are cleansing the head, eyes and fatigue. Repeat 8 times or more.

2.   Breathe in and visualize the universal Qi coming down, reaching your crown, flowing into your head. Breathe out and move the energy down to come out of the chest centre (2). As the energy flows, visualize it cleansing the entire pathway. Repeat 8 times or more.

3.   Breathe in and visualize the universal Qi coming down, reaching your crown, flowing into your head. Breathe out and move the energy flow down to come out of the lower abdominal centre (3). As the energy flows, visualize you are cleansing the entire pathway of chest, abdominal and organs as it leaves you. Repeat 8 times or more. Like a river, chi flows.

4.   Breathe in and visualize universal Qi coming down, reaching your crown, flowing into your head. Breathe out and continue to move the energy and allow it to flow down to the ground and into the earth. Repeat 8 times or more. Relax and breathe.

Building Chi between the Palm of Your Hands

Recharging our battery can be just this simple. While Chi Gong forms are easiest to learn with an instructor, please recognize the importance of deliberate breaths and visualization. It is also helpful to cultivate Chi between your hands. Hold a ball of energy, or Chi, that feels as light as a cloud between the palms of your hands. With your palms facing each other, place them a foot-length apart. Widen and close your hands with your breath. Slowly, you will feel the energy of magnetism or warmth. This is healing Chi.

Chi Gong in Canada

Many people also use Qi Gong practice for increasing DHEA, reducing stress and addressing specific health issues such as shortness of breath, fatigue, fibromyalgia, pain, digestive problems, diabetes, blood pressure issues, headaches and autoimmune problems. It is particularly important to note there is actually a Qi Gong exercise designed for vision. In 1990, my teacher, Grand Master Wu, led a team of 100 healthcare professionals on Wu's Eye Qi Gong® research studies and went through 4,000 medical research studies in China. The same studies were repeated for three years with the same 4,000 participants and had a proven success rate of over 90 percent! We have brought this Chi Gong to Canada in Toronto.

The Wu's Eye Qi Gong form is now used to support the healing of all kinds of eye problems: fatigue, pain, headaches, migraines and insomnia and is also an immune booster.

The Chi energy is positive. Once you practice it for a time, you will feel different from how you did before your practice. It removes ill thoughts and fatigue. As you feel lighter, you have much more room for compassion and kindness. Your strength returns, bringing back your passion for life. As you are lighter, you can see your new pathway, which may have been shadowed before. The practice of Qi Gong helps you get to the point of self-actualization.

The physical heart is the organ, which fails more often than
any other. Heart Chi Gong is a masterful approach for releasing
the cumulative psychological trauma underlying all heart disease.
C. Normal Shealy, MD, PhD, Founder and CEO of the
International Institute of Holistic Medicine

If you have read to this point, you may find it most interesting to know more about how Qi Gong can unclutter difficult emotions and promote detachment. This is covered extensively in my second book, the number-one international bestseller, Unlocking Your Happiness Within: Living the Life You Choose with Chi Gong. The book and workbook are available on Amazon:
http://getbook.at/UnlockingYourHappinessWithin.

My first book, Life Force: The Miraculous Power of Qi Gong, helps readers understand what Chi gong is and its power to heal. It is filled with inspirational stories of students who overcame physical and/or emotional challenges to transform their lives.

I only ask you to be open-minded and give yourself a chance. The next time you feel tired, be kind to yourself and practice a few breaths. You will feel rejuvenated and recharge your battery. I would be happy to show you how to do this.

How Did I Discover Chi Gong?

As a young person, when I was twenty, I was seriously ill with tuberculosis. All my life I had had to seek out how to heal myself. I became a single mother twenty-some years ago, raising children aged eleven, six and five. Qi Gong has played an important role in my life, giving me energy, rebalancing me physically and emotionally as I worked through some of the biggest stresses of life with limited resources. Chi Gong gave me courage and much love. Like all teachers, I teach what I have learned in my life.

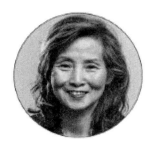

About
Master Teresa Yeung

Master Teresa Yeung is an internationally recognized Master of Chi Gong, healer and # 1 international bestselling author who speaks on how to achieve physical, emotional and spiritual balance with Chi Gong.

She is the founder of Pureland International Qi Gong and The Seventh Happiness® School of Chi Gong, a certified private institution. She is the sole successor of Grand Master Weizhao Wu's lineage. Wu, a distinguished Chi Gong master, educator and creator of the highly successful Wu's Eye Qi Gong, helped millions of people.

Yeung is also approved by the USA National Certification Commission for Acupuncturists and Oriental Medicine (NCCAOM) as a continuing education professional development activity (PDA) provider.

Great blessings!

For more information, visit:
www.purelandqigong.com
www.facebook.com/purelandqigong/

New Online Live Program:
Fa Chi Gong Instructor Online Live Certification Program - learn to teach, heal and practice Fa Chi (send Chi) in 3 months

Chapter 20
Essential Life Lessons Learned Through Pageantry

By: Ms. Divya Sieudarsan

Before pageantry, I hadn't realized how unexciting my life was. My life was spent in work and school and there wasn't a future for me besides more work after I finished school. I was taking the path everyone took: trying to figure out by the end of high school what I wanted to do for the rest of my life, go to college or university to learn how to do it and then, hopefully, find an excellent, well-paying job I could use those skills in.

That is great for some people; it is their life's dream, but I came to understand I wanted more and it showed up out of the blue one day.

A scout at my university happened to see me playing table tennis. He came up to me and said, "Hey, have you ever thought of doing pageants?"

"No way." I was a tomboy and pageantry was the last thing on my mind. That was for girly girls, so I laughed it off. I had no respect for it at all.

Unfazed, he said, "Here's my card with my number. Give me a call if you're interested. I see a lot of potential in you."

I went back and told my friends and we all had a good laugh.

When I went home and told my family, they said, "Well, if this is something you want to do, you should do it."

Something in me clicked. I remembered my grandfather and I used to watch Miss Universe together when I was small. He would say, "I'm going to sign you up for one of these pageants." We would laugh about it.

Now, for the first time, I thought I should give it a try for the fun of it. I signed up and got into my first pageant. I didn't win—it was one of those sad experiences, but that didn't stop me. I got into another; I was a runner up, but still no crown. I eventually captured a title and ended up in a major international competition. Even though I didn't win, it changed my life and I am so thankful.

When I got into pageants, I realized it takes so much more than what was on the outside of me.

First, you need to have so much confidence in yourself, to project it outward for other people to see. If you are in a shell, you are not going to relate to the crowd, or they are not going to see what you have to offer.

Pageantry opens up a whole new world for you. You get to network with many people, including very influential ones like presidents, ministers and successful entrepreneurs and through them opportunities arise. If the president or minister needed a new member of staff and you had the qualifications and presented yourself appropriately, then guess what? You may have just landed an interview or a recommendation. Opportunities are sometimes disguised and some are in plain sight.

The world of charity opened up to me as well. I got to see first-hand how people struggle and why these charities are so important. My heart broke when we went to a home for kids who were hiding from the abusers who hurt them. My position now afforded me the ability to fundraise and help these essential programs.

Getting In Shape Wasn't As Easy As I Thought

One place I struggled the most was physically preparing for the pageants themselves. For the international pageant, I had only two months to prepare. The organization gave me a personal trainer. Every single day after work I would do laps, then we would do exercises—a full three hours of training or more. Weekends also, because I had to get in shape.

I also had to eat healthy, because my trainer said, "You can work out as much as you can, but as long as you don't eat right, it's not going to help." I was a junk-food-aholic.

At work we had a cook who would prepare delicious food daily and lots of treats—everything I wasn't supposed to eat. Then in the evenings, when we worked late, we would order in burgers, fries and all sorts of fast foods. They were temptations I had to learn to conquer.

Because it was such a short time I went on a strict diet. Just water, no soda, no tea, no juices. Strictly baked foods, nothing fried. My protein was chicken and fish: just baked chicken or fish with vegetables on the side. I would sneak in a little mashed potato every once in a while. The commitment showed fast results because of the exercise and the diet combined. I stayed away from diet pills and non-holistic methods since I am conscious of the side effects of these drugs.

My schedule was also crazy. I would do interviews in addition to my work. So, I would go get my hair and my make-up done and then do the interview, many times on my lunch or dinner break. I was determined to succeed and I did.

Of course, now I am not on such a strict diet. I eat freely, but I am more conscious about my health. If I continue eating junk food all the time, how is it going to affect me? Diabetes runs in my family. I've watched my grandfather inject himself with insulin on a daily basis and witnessed how Diabetes robbed him of bits and pieces of his life until the end. I realized that healthy eating and exercise needed to become part of my lifestyle if I wanted to live a long healthy life.

For a more in depth look on Diabetes, be sure to read Cheryl's chapter.

What I Learned from Pageantry That Will Help You

I didn't know it at the time, but my experiences in the pageants were preparing me to be successful in life. I want to share with you the most important ones that not only helped me, but will help you as well.

Coaching

I was a procrastinator and would do things at the last minute, but I soon realized that is not how you accomplish anything in life. My coach pushed me and reminded me that if I didn't do what I need to do then, I won't see any results later. She helped me to see the consequences of my actions, which motivated me to keep moving forward.

My personal trainer would only let me take ten-second breaks while I was exercising. I wanted to take half an hour! This showed me I was capable of so much more than I thought. When she pushed me beyond my self-imposed limits, I became more than what I thought possible. You need someone with an outside perspective to push yet guide you on a better path.

A coach will also help you to accomplish your goals faster. What would have taken me six months took only two with her. She prepared me not only to physically be on stage, but mentally too. A good coach never just helps you in one area of life, but in all of them.

How to Lose Weight and Get in Shape Quickly and Safely

One of the biggest things that helped me was increasing my water intake and decrease all other forms of liquid. In our Caribbean society we are unaware of how many calories we consume by drinking soda, alcohol and fancy caffeinated drinks. Just by cutting out one can of cola a day you will lose, or at least not gain, almost seventeen pounds in a year. Just imagine what will happen when you cut out most of the other drinks as well.

Also, most people are in a slightly dehydrated state, which causes the body not to function at optimal efficiency. By increasing your water intake, you increase your metabolism and mental function, making it easier for you to lose weight.

Stick to your diet! For fast results you must avoid all unhealthy food, even a bite. List your do's and don'ts and do not navigate. You must be determined to get your desired results.

Give yourself a mental plan. What I mean is you must decide how you are going to handle temptation before it comes. What are you going to tell yourself that will convince you not to eat that bad food? For me, I would say to myself, "If I want to see these results, I need to give this up for at least right now."

How to Show Confidence No Matter Where You Go

Confidence is something you have to build. For me that meant reading a lot and becoming versatile in many subjects so wherever I go, whatever topic comes up, I know I can answer any question or be able to engage in the conversation. I also learned when I didn't know about a topic, it was okay to ask questions. I learned how to do it in such a way that I still came across as confident.

How to Stay Healthy While Travelling

Confidence has to do with believing in yourself. When you do, it projects outward and others see it. Whatever you are thinking in your mind mentally, how you prepare yourself mentally, that's the type of energy you exude.

This can be very hard, especially for me. When I go on vacation, I find there are all-you-can-eat buffets for breakfast, lunch and dinner. I want to indulge as much as possible and sometimes I do, but I have also learned to control myself. At the buffets I focus on the fruits and vegetables and stick to water every day.

I also put exercise in when I travel. Which can be very hard, because you have to schedule it, or you have to wake up earlier, or go to bed later; it takes a lot of determination. But again, once you have that goal in mind you make it happen. Like you do every other day, you have to make conscious choices about what you put into your mouth and keeping yourself active.

How to Win Without the Crown?

For a more in-depth focus on staying healthy while travelling, take a look at Charles' chapter.

The concept behind this is that although you didn't win the crown, you gained so much more in the process. Me, I accumulated many followers who look up to me as a role model, I became a voice that could help impact our communities and make the world a little better by spreading positivity. Of course, I won't forget the knowledge and experience that I passed on to others.

There wasn't time to mope or be sad, because I started working towards making a positive impact. I also had a great impact on young women who come to me for advice. Value was added to my community and I was able to make more of a difference which I had not been able to do before.

I went to different orphanages, spending time with the children there. Just being there for someone means you can actually help mould people into better human beings. I became a different person and I liked who I was.

This also applies to you. How do you deal with life when you didn't win the prize, or the job went to someone else? Those are moments that define you and determine your future. You can choose to put yourself into a tailspin or you can look at the positive. You have to think, "Okay, I didn't get it this time and there was a reason for that." I believe everything happens in its own time and everything happens for a reason.

I feel if you did not get that promotion or the contract or whatever the case is, it has to do with something bigger. Maybe it's not your time. Maybe you need to prepare a little more. Maybe you need to build a little more confidence in yourself. Maybe you need to put a little more work into this and try again.

You have to have a positive frame of mind. Don't just knock yourself down and say, "I'm a loser. I didn't get it." That is the worst thing you can do to yourself, because your self-worth is never based on winning.

How to Stay True to Yourself

In pageantry and life, it is easy to get carried away with what people expect you to be.

I would watch previous queens, how they behave, their personality and would be tempted to be just like them. I learned everyone has a unique personality. Everyone has a unique way to shine.

While it may work for you, it may not work for me. I feel no matter what, although you are preparing and doing these things to refine yourself, you still need to be true to you. Bring your personality out. Make sure all of these things aren't overshadowing who you really are.

When you are on a platform or even at a job, whatever it is, stand your ground, stay true to yourself in the aspect of what your belief is and what you see as being right.

It is okay for you to be you. You were created the way you are for a reason. You are unique and wonderfully made. There is no one else exactly like you and there never will be, so celebrate it. Rejoice in who you are. Find your purpose and never let anyone talk you out of it.

You Can Become More

The biggest lesson I learned and I want to share with you, is you can become more than you even imagined. Les Brown says there is greatness inside of you waiting to come out. I am so thankful that scout saw potential in me and gave me the chance to become the real me. The pageant queen waiting to come out.

Living your dream is not always easy. It is going to take hard work and patience. You are going to have to sacrifice to see the real you come forth, but when it does, you will be so happy and it will be worth everything you had to give up to get there.

I would love to connect with you. Find me on Facebook "Divya Sieudarsan" and let's take the next step together. To the Queen or King in all of us.

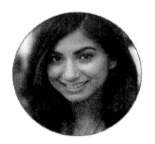

About
Ms. Divya Sieudarsan

Ms. Divya Sieudarsan was born in Guyana, South America. She has experience on stage, on the mic and the catwalk. Divya isn't just a pretty smile, she's a positively motivated individual who has represented Guyana internationally as Miss India Guyana in 2014. Divya has worked with organizations and volunteers across Guyana to make a difference. She believes through positivity and awareness, we can get to the root of the issues and work it out bit by bit.

Divya jumped into entrepreneurship at the age of 22. Apart from being a marketing consultant, she also has vast experience and knowledge in accounting, aviation, customer service, human resources, sales, training and management. As a marketing consultant, she works with clients globally, mainly in North and South America.

Divya has worked with many underprivileged individuals and communities, she wants to help improve the lives of those who are in unfortunate circumstances and those having second thoughts about living this beautiful life God created. Divya hopes to motivate each individual to realize the power of positivity and upliftment in every aspect of life. Positive energy can overcome all hardships and lead to a healthier, happier and wealthier life.

About Local Experts Group

LocalExperts™
People Building Our Community

Partnership Opportunity

Our vision is to help you create and distribute authentic and reputable content. Our mission is to donate $1 for every book sold to feeding and educating children in underserved regions worldwide.

As this book is about Health, Wealth and Happiness, we would like to share with you how to be apart of this expert's community. So, you can also do exactly what each of these 21 authors are already doing. That is to share their knowledge, expertise and skills with the world and leave a legacy that will remain even after we are all gone.

If you enjoyed the content and layout of this book and would like to collaborate in an upcoming "The Handbook to ™" book series, or be a Brand Ambassador of, or an Affiliate for Local Experts Group, be sure to contact us at: **www.localexpertsgroup.com or call 1-647-919-8131**.

We love working with individuals who are experts, coaches, mentors, speakers, authors, trainers, teachers, promoters and anyone in sales who have a desire to become a published author and create online and DVD courses to add value to your audience.

We work with religious organizations world-wide to help your leaders create and publish materials to reach a wider audience which creates an avenue for fund-raising opportunities.

We work with Corporations, NGO, Non-profits - whether large or small and Government agencies to publish promotional, commemorative and collaborative publications.

CEO and Co-founder,
Raymond Harlall